The Real Fountain of Youth

Simple Lifestyle Changes for Productive Longevity

Eraldo Maglara

with Stacy Reagan and Mary Ellen Landolfi

CONTENTS

FOREWORD

When Eraldo and I first discussed his plans for a book on athletic training and productive longevity, I was immediately excited. Training is a continuing part of my life physically and mentally. First, as a physician I continue to expand and adapt my practice of medicine as science and learning afford the opportunity. Second, as an "athlete" I continue to train my body to live life to its fullest and adapt to life as I grow older. I consider us all potential athletes in one way or another, whether through a physical hobby or an actual sport. The essence of athleticism is improving our physical performance. Having goals and enjoying accomplishment in physical activity helps sustain us and complements our more purely mental pursuits.

I have found that the benefits of athletic training improve when I have a teacher or trainer helping me. Trying to identify how this works can be separated into technical guidance, motivation, and planning skills given by a trainer. When I was training for a triathlon, my trainer began by helping me with my running stride and swimming stroke. He also had a training schedule mapped out for daily workouts. Finally, after logging my results for the week, he would review and offer critiques to help me improve.

What is not as obvious is what a trainer prevents. I see the problems caused by overtraining and injuries on a daily basis in my office. Many of these injuries are avoidable. Through smarter training, a trainer improves our performance by helping to keep us focused and avoiding time spent rehabilitating injuries.

This book will be a welcome guide and inspiration for people looking to increase or improve their health and well being through athletic training. Eraldo took on the task of simplifying tedious manuals of exercises and incorporating insights from other professionals to produce an intriguing and inspiring guide to becoming and staying fit and content. He highlights the

1

benefits of a true athletic trainer in helping us achieve these goals. Having seen both Eraldo's practice and his philosophy as an athletic trainer develop over the years that I have known him, I commend him on sharing his knowledge with us in this book.

Steven P. Lisser, MD
Chairman, Department of Orthopaedics
Riverview Medical Center

CHAPTER 2

Longevity Is Up To You

A few years ago, a good friend of mine told me his mother was having knee surgery. Days later, after a successful operation, his mom was recovering at a rehabilitation facility and receiving physical therapy. I stopped by to visit and to see if she had any questions I could answer or if there was anything I could do for her. At that moment, a nurse came in and we were told to wait outside. I couldn't help but notice that the majority of people there were senior citizens, and that many of them showed no obvious signs of physical limitations.

I struck up a conversation with one of the attending nurses. "It seems to me that most people here don't have anything physically wrong. Is that correct?" I asked. She reflected for a moment, then said "Getting old is just a part of life."

No—it is not! I want to assure you that you do not have to simply surrender to old age. It is possible to maintain most, if not all, of your strength and flexibility as you grow older. "Getting old" in the sense of slowing down, becoming feeble and giving up being active is a decision that you make mentally. The physical changes and limitations that people experience as old age are just their bodies following the mental command and responding to the lack of use.

That event changed everything for me. And the more I thought about it, the more I realized that I could start training, teaching, energizing these people. I could give them motivation and confidence. And more importantly, I now had a mission—to show people that the sad acceptance of aging and its lack of mobility and independence is not inevitable. You can stay productive as you age. How? Through movement, through diet, through mindset.

I'm sure you're not surprised by the first two components. To paraphrase Newton's First Law of Motion: a body in motion tends to stay in motion—and that is true of the human body as well. In general, the more active you are as you get older, the more active you tend to stay. This is true in part because staying active becomes a habit. And you can cultivate that habit to make activity a seamless and continuous part of your life.

Diet is also an important factor, and one that we are all aware of. Fresh, quality food fuels your body more efficiently and more effectively than pre-packaged, processed food. We know that—we've all heard it multiple times, from multiple sources, but the perception is that it's easier and quicker to grab a box or open a can than to prepare something from scratch. Numerous companies have spent a lot of marketing dollars to convince us of that, but with a little preparation and planning you can make some important changes in your diet that will result in a healthier you.

The last, and perhaps the most important component, is you. Your outlook, the mindset you have about your health and longevity, is perhaps the most important aspect of all. Yes, you can do things right now to help yourself live a longer, more productive life. But there is no quick fix. Although there are entire industries out there promoting this pill or that device to give you a beach-ready body, they rarely deliver a lasting, permanent change. But if your goal is a productive longevity, then your mind needs to be focused on that, and you need to be willing and even eager to do a little bit every day to get there.

It will take work to become healthier and more active, but it does not have to be a chore. It's all a matter of how you look at it. Focusing on how much better you feel each day, and reconnecting to the world around you can be very motivating. Choosing instead to complain about having to spend time every day exercising and moping about the entire bag of potato chips you can no longer eat will defeat you before you even get started. Staying productive as you age is certainly possible, but you are going to have to get up off the couch to get there.

CHAPTER 3

Why Start Now?

Every minute of every day we are getting older. How happy we are with that fact depends on what mile marker we happen to be standing next to on the highway of life. Someone who has just turned 50 will not typically anticipate a birthday as much as someone approaching 21. But, until the day we die, time marches on for all of us. We can't stop it.

But we can, however, slow many of the effects that we have come to believe are synonymous with aging. Decreased mobility and balance problems, osteoporosis, spinal curvatures, dietary problems, intolerances and restrictions, lack of stamina, depression, and the numerous aches and pains that seem to increase every year—many of these can be avoided by staying active, watching your diet and keeping a positive outlook.

Genetics does play a part, but physical changes related to aging are by no means set in stone. Many people who have been active and remain active as they grow older show fewer outward signs of aging. Think Jamie Lee Curtis, Chuck Norris, Bruce Springsteen, Lauren Hutton and the incomparable Betty White. While Betty isn't talking, the rest all readily admit that they adhere to some sort of regular physical activity.

Need more convincing? Below is a short list of the most common age-related changes:

- hearing impairment
- vision changes
- arthritis

- hypertension

- heart disease

- diabetes

- osteoporosis

- mental and cognitive changes

- memory loss

- difficulty with everyday tasks

While some of these ailments result from genetic factors or cumulative damage over a lifetime, many can be lessened, alleviated or possibly avoided altogether by a targeted exercise plan and attention to diet. Disease aside, performing daily tasks gets more difficult as people get older. Studies show that just under ten percent of people aged 65 to 69 require personal assistance with everyday activities. By age 85, however, that number increases to 50 percent. Half of all people 85 and older will need help accomplishing daily tasks.

That means out of every two people, one will need help caring for themselves. If you are married, that's you or your spouse—statistically, one of you gets to be a caregiver or personal assistant for the other. And all "old-married-couple" jokes aside, that's a lot of pressure to place on a loved one, especially when there are things you can do to avoid it.

In an article entitled "Aging: What to Expect" The Mayo Clinic details changes in your body's various systems and explains things you can do to counter these changes. While the bodily changes run from high blood pressure to urinary incontinence to memory loss and brittle, porous bones, exercise and dietary changes are among the recommended actions to prevent or relieve nearly every condition on the list.

Why the urgency? Much like investing money for retirement, the sooner you start laying the groundwork for a healthy future, the better your outcome. In this case, you will have fewer bad habits to break and hopefully less damage to undo. Study after study has shown that participating in physical activity can enhance the quality of life into advanced old age, and can help stave off some degenerative diseases and even some chronic illnesses. The sooner you start, the sooner you begin to make positive changes to your body. And that translates into having more energy and stamina, being more flexible, more confident and yes, just overall feeling better.

Currently, the average life expectancy for a man is about 76 years, 81 years for a woman. The average life expectancy has increased steadily over the past few hundred years, due to changes in nutrition, sanitation and medicine among other things. It is worth pointing out, however, that while rates are rising overall, what used to be a significant gap between life expectancies for men and for women is shrinking as women are succumbing to higher rates of heart disease, cancer and stress-related diseases.

The question to ask yourself is: How do you want to spend those extra years? Doing all those things you always wanted to do? Playing with your grandkids? Vacationing with your spouse? Being able to walk up a flight of stairs? Or being confined to a wheelchair adjusting to the fact of getting older? I think the choice is pretty simple.

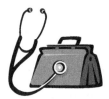

More Facts

Just in case the previous section didn't convince you, I've included some more studies. I want you to understand that exercise—keeping your body in shape and in motion can't be something you put off until you have time or until you have an issue. Like investing, the sooner you begin, the better your results. Below are a few more reasons why you should start today. All of the information below is from reliable sources, and all the links are listed in the Footnotes section of this book. I encourage you to do more research on your own and to discuss this information with your doctor.

The need to stay active as we age is nothing new. Decades ago, in a 1979 report entitled *Healthy People: The Surgeon General's Report on Health Promotion and Disease Prevention*, the Surgeon General noted: "As do younger people, older Americans hope for a state of well-being which would allow them to perform at their highest functional capacity on physical, psychological, and social levels. Their greatest fear is of being helpless, useless, sick, or unable to care for themselves."[3]

Let's address some of the more common ailments that become an issue as people get older, and the impact those conditions can have on a person's health and independence.

Breaking a Hip: People in my parents' and grandparents' generation lived in fear of breaking a hip. As it turns out, the older generations were not wrong in equating falling and breaking a hip with dying. Here is a quote from Richard Carmona, in his 2004 Surgeon General's Report on bone health:

> From an individual's perspective, bone disease has a devastating impact on patients and their families. While few die directly from bone disease, for many individuals a fracture can lead to a downward spiral in physical and mental health that for some ultimately results in death. In fact, hip fractures are associated with a significantly increased risk of death, especially during the first year after the fracture.[4]

According to the Centers for Disease Control, a large proportion of fall deaths are due to complications following a hip fracture. One out of five hip fracture patients dies within a year of their injury. Up to one in four adults who lived independently before their hip fracture remains in a nursing home for at least a year after their injury.[5]

Along with these frightening statistics the CDC offers some advice for prevention. Not surprisingly their tips to avoid the debilitating snowball effect of breaking a hip are centered around fall prevention. Their recommendations include:

- Exercise regularly
- Promote strength, flexibility and balance training
- Review medicines to eliminate dizziness
- Remove trip hazards and add safety improvements in your home
- Get sufficient calcium and Vitamin D in your diet[6]

Diabetes: Diabetes is basically having too much sugar in your blood. Whether that is due to a problem with insulin or some other factor, Type 2 diabetes, which used to be called non-insulin-dependent diabetes mellitus or adult-onset diabetes, is a very serious problem. "Diabetes can cause serious health complications including heart disease, blindness, kidney failure, and lower-extremity amputations. Diabetes is the seventh leading cause of death in the United States."[7]

Fortunately, for many people Type 2 diabetes can be delayed if not avoided altogether. The primary issue with diabetes is managing blood sugar levels, and the simplest way to do that is by exercising and eating properly.

The Centers for Disease have a lot of information regarding diabetes on their website. In response to the question "Can diabetes be prevented?" they say: "A number of studies have shown that regular physical activity can significantly reduce the risk of developing Type 2 diabetes. Type 2 diabetes is associated with obesity."[8]

Under a section devoted to information on preventing diabetes, they post another question and an even more detailed response:

What are the most important things to do to prevent diabetes?
 The Diabetes Prevention Program (DPP), a major federally funded study of 3,234 people at high risk for diabetes, showed that people can delay and possibly prevent the disease by losing a small amount of weight (5 to 7 percent of total body weight) through 30 minutes of physical activity 5 days a week and healthier eating.[9]

Heart Disease: In the longest running study on aging, the National Institute on Aging's (NIA) Baltimore Longitudinal Study of Aging (BLSA) has given us a look at aging by following a broad range of people for over 50 years. Founded to determine what normal aging looked like, this study showed that age-related changes "do not inevitably lead to diseases such as diabetes, hypertension, or dementia. A number of disorders that typically occur in old age are a result of disease processes, not normal aging."[10]

Heart disease, a problem for many older adults, may also be alleviated by exercise. Scientists have long known that regular exercise causes certain changes in the hearts of younger people. These changes, which include lowering resting heart rate and increasing heart mass and stroke volume (the amount of blood pumped with each heart beat), make the heart a better pump. Evidence now suggests that people who begin exercise training in later life, for instance in their sixties and seventies, can also experience improved heart function.

In one study, BLSA researchers observed a decrease in the risk of a coronary event, like a heart attack, in older male BLSA participants who took part in high intensity, leisure time physical activity like lap swimming or running.[11]

Alzheimer's Disease / Dementia - Cognitive problems are also a big concern as people get older, and dementia or Alzheimer's disease can quickly derail your plans and eliminate your independence. While we still don't know a lot about what causes these issues, some preliminary research is showing that your brain, like any other muscle, needs to remain active to stay healthy. Because your brain handles so many complex functions, it appears that a mix of academic, social and physical activities can help stave off cognitive woes.

We have this from the BLSA study: "People who are involved in hobbies and social and leisure activities may be at lower risk for some health problems. For example, one study followed participants for up to 21 years and linked leisure activities, like reading, playing board games, playing musical instruments, and dancing, with a lower risk for dementia."[12]

The National Institute on Aging has a report titled "Preventing Alzheimer's Disease: What Do We Know?" They note that "Epidemiological studies and some intervention studies suggest that physical exercise may also play a role in reducing risk for Alzheimer's disease and age-related cognitive decline."[13]

Based on animal studies, researchers speculate that exercise causes increased blood flow in the brain and this strengthens and the blood vessels and the nerve connections there. Some recent studies also think exercise may be responsible for higher levels of a protein called nerve growth factor, which is important for memory and learning.[14]

In a year-long study, 65 older people exercised daily, doing either an aerobic exercise program of walking for 40 minutes or a nonaerobic program of stretching and toning exercises. At the end of the trial, the walking group showed improved connectivity in the part of the brain engaged in daydreaming, envisioning the future, and recalling the past. The walking group also improved on executive function, the ability to plan and organize tasks such as cooking a meal.[15]

Following a healthy diet plan also plays a role in preventing cognitive decline. The NIA states:

> Studies have found, for example, that a diet rich in vegetables, especially green leafy vegetables and cruciferous vegetables like broccoli, is associated with a reduced rate of cognitive decline. One epidemiological study reported that people who ate a "Mediterranean diet" had a 28 percent lower risk of developing MCI (mild cognitive impairment) and a 48 percent lower risk of progressing from MCI to Alzheimer's disease.[16]

So, despite the dire forecasts, there is hope. Discussing the health of older Americans, Surgeon General Julius B. Richmond in 1979 went on to note that "... many measures can be applied to increase independence, self-sufficiency and quality of life for the elderly."[17]

One last quote from Dr. Richmond, who was way ahead of his time, discussing productive longevity long before the phrase was even coined:

> Exercise and fitness for older people need emphasis. Aging is not—or should not—be a process of mere passivity. Nor should the obsolescent image of inevitable incapacitation be allowed to continue. Movement is part of functional living—and the quality of intellectual and physical performance is enhanced by remaining or becoming physically fit in old age.[18]

Human beings are made to be active, and continued physical activity enables you to remain active as you age. As the above studies show, the repercussions of inactivity and poor diet can be serious. I'm sure many of you have done some form of financial planning for your retirement. So too, you need to do some physical planning for your "golden years." It's never too late to start.

I'll close this chapter with another quote from the BLSA study:

> In fact, exercise and physical activity are considered a cornerstone to almost every healthy aging program. Emerging scientific evidence suggests that people who exercise regularly not only live longer, they live better. And, being physically active —

doing everyday activities that keep your body moving such as gardening, walking the dog, and taking the stairs instead of the elevator — can help you to continue to do the things you enjoy and stay independent as you age.

Specifically, regular exercise and physical activity can reduce your risk of developing some diseases and disabilities that often occur with age. For instance, balance exercises help prevent falls, a major cause of disability in older adults. Strength exercises build muscles and reduce the risk of osteoporosis. Flexibility or stretching exercises help keep your body limber and give you the freedom of movement you need to do your everyday activities.[19]

I couldn't have said it better myself.

you've seen in Chapter 3, studies have shown that in many cases there is a disturbingly short period of time between a broken hip and death in elderly patients. What the studies don't show is why this correlation exists. As with anything, there are several reasons, but I believe there are two main items at work here: first, the injury causes them to stop moving, and second, they begin to think of themselves as "disabled," and often, they just give up.

We all know of someone in the generation above ours who was petrified of falling and breaking a hip, because they knew people who went into the hospital with a broken hip and never came out. This fear of dying from a broken hip becomes a self-fulfilling prophecy—and yes, the fact that the person fell, that their bones were brittle enough that they broke a hip, perhaps they were alone and had to wait a long time for help, all bespeak underlying medical issues—but we can't discount the impact of a person's beliefs. If you are absolutely convinced that you will die because you fell and broke your hip, the odds become far greater that you will do so.

I am going to show you how to channel the strength of your mind to help support positive changes in your life. In the next few chapters you will learn some basic yet effective exercises that will help you remain flexible and keep your muscles strong. You will read nutritional advice to help you make healthy choices in the way you eat. You will learn about the way your body functions and get some pointers on how to make sure all your systems work together efficiently. And you will understand that these changes can make a big difference in the way you feel today, and more importantly, in the way you will feel tomorrow and all the tomorrows after.

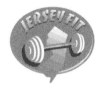

CHAPTER 5

Getting Started

Prior to beginning any journey, a person must do two things. You need to create a map of where you are going, and you need to pack for your trip. Easy, you say, I want productive longevity. Fine—wonderful really, because wanting to get there is a good chunk of the struggle. But not even Mapquest™ can guide you to your destination if you don't know where you are starting from.

We are not going to spend a lot of time filling out questionnaires or charting where you are right now, but you do need to have a clear idea of where you are so that you can see your progress. Achievement is a very motivating factor!

Also, you will need a plan—the steps you will follow to achieve your goal. Bear in mind that productive longevity is, by its very nature, a moving target. It is a lifestyle you work towards, not a goal you achieve and then forget about. Over the next few chapters you will find the steps to start your journey towards a healthier lifestyle. While any exercise will help you get into shape, for optimum health, you can't just run or only lift weights. The key will be to incorporate a variety of physical activity into your life, so that you can continue to be physically active as you get older.

There are many ways to be active. You can be active in short spurts throughout the day or you can set aside specific times of the day or specific days of the week to exercise. Many physical activities, such as brisk walking or raking leaves, are free or low-cost and do not require special equipment.[21]

27

The above quote is from the BLSA study on aging, and notice they never once say that you have to go to the gym! I think by now you realize that getting active and staying active is something you really must do, not only for yourself but also for your loved ones. Physical activity is every bit as important as you get older as it is to have life insurance or a will. If you are a person who hates working out, it may be every bit as onerous, but in the long run, the rewards of feeling better and maintaining your independence are perhaps even more essential.

Introduction to Fitness Training

Do you hate to exercise? Don't feel bad, you are not alone. The key is to figure out why you hate to exercise—is it too boring? Are the movements too difficult? Do you hate to get up early? Are you too tired at night? Be honest with yourself about what you dislike and what is keeping you from getting started. Nothing is etched in stone, and everything is customizable. Don't like to work out first thing? There are many reasons to schedule your daily workout early in the day, but if that doesn't work than by all means pencil it in during the afternoon or later. If you dislike going to the gym, or you hate sports, try dance or yoga as your activity instead.

Ideally, you should schedule the exercise program that I give in Chapter 9 into your daily routine. The program will flex and strengthen all your major muscle groups, but it is designed for you to work every group twice a week. I do not expect you to do the entire routine, start to finish, every day! Break it into pieces—one day work your upper body, the next day work your core, etc. Do 10 minutes in the morning while you are waiting for your coffee, 10 minutes before or after lunch, 10 minutes before bed—whatever works! Of course, if you can only find time twice a week to exercise, then go ahead and perform the entire sequence.

And while you certainly need to focus on increasing your flexibility and building strength, cardio is important as well. For that reason it is essential that you find ways to increase your activity level as part of your everyday life. Remember, the more you do, the more you will be able to do, and the easier it will be to move, to bend, to lift things.

If you are afraid of exercising because you always seem to get hurt, you need to be sure to start off the right way. First and foremost, check with your doctor to see if you have issues that would prevent you from exercising. Ask your doctor if there are any movements he or she recommends that you avoid. Show them this book, discuss with them the exercises that I describe in Chapter 9. Talk to them about any questions you have after reading the Nutrition or Chiropractic sections. Your doctor is a professional that you hire to assist you in maintaining your health—he or she should not only be aware of this change you are making, but should also be a part of your support team. Perhaps more than anyone else, your doctor is aware of the current state of your health—it is important to consult him or her to be certain they do not have any restrictions for you, or wish to see you modify any movement.

Make sure you are doing the exercises properly. Your body has to be challenged, your muscles have to be worked nearly to their limit in order to become stronger, but I cannot stress enough how important it is to make sure you have the correct form. Doing any exercise improperly can engage muscles that are not targeted or you can end up working a muscle beyond its range of motion—both of which can result in an injury.

I don't want to see you sidelined before you really get started. Even life-long exercise fans can be put off by an injury. And yet, achieving and maintaining proper form throughout a series of exercises can be a challenge. To be absolutely certain that you are keeping the correct form when exercising, the ideal situation would be to hire a Personal Trainer, either privately or at a gym, to supervise as you work through your routine for the first few times. For many people, unfortunately, that is not an option, so I have tried to be as clear and specific as possible in my exercise descriptions. I will also be uploading videos to my websites— www.TheRealFountainOfYouthBook.com or www.JerseyFitTV.com— which will demonstrate many of the exercises given in Chapter 9.

Sometimes, even if you are performing the exercises correctly and you have perfect form, something can feel off. I don't mean just difficult, I mean something feels like it isn't moving easily or there is some pain with a certain movement. This can signal an underlying problem. To address just such a situation, in Chapter 11, I have interviewed two Chiropractic professionals to address your body's alignment and how proper alignment can enhance your performance and your health.

Where Am I Now?

Although I said earlier that we won't spend much time on a current assessment, it is important to know what your fitness level is right now. This matters for two reasons. First, a current assessment will help in designing your routine. If the most active thing you've done this week is pick up this book, you are not to attempt to run a mile-and-a-half tomorrow. I know you are impatient to see results, but too much too fast will result in soreness and possibly even injury. Be honest with yourself about your current state, so that you can plan a fitness routine that works for you, and that you can continue to work long after the novelty has worn off.

Second, knowing what your current fitness levels are allows you to track your progress. There will be progress! The scale might not reflect it right away, but you might notice that your clothes fit better. Since muscle actually weighs more than fat, you may not see any change in weight, and yet your groceries may be easier to carry or you might notice that you don't have to catch your breath after climbing the stairs. These are all signs of progress and they all count! I want you to track these changes so that you can see what you are achieving, and know that it is worthwhile to continue the program.

Following is a very simple chart—you know if you spend all of your free time in front of the television—I won't ask you to write that here. But this chart will help you note some specifics that will let you know where you are starting from today. I will include another copy of this chart at the end of the book so that you can track your progress. I suggest that you check yourself every month or two—even when you do not see progress in one aspect, such as weight loss, you will usually see gains in strength or endurance.

Another excellent gauge of strength is a yoga position called the Plank. The Plank is a position that utilizes the muscles in your core, but many muscle groups will be engaged to maintain it, which is why it is such a wonderful movement to track your progress. Instructions on how to do the Plank are included in Chapter 9, but in short to do the Plank, get into the "up" position for a push up—and hold it! Use a stopwatch to time how long you can stay in the Plank, and write that time down. I guarantee as you get more fit, the amount of time you can hold a Plank will increase as well.

Progress is motivating! When you see how far you've come, you will want to achieve even more!

Initial Self-Assessment of Fitness Levels

Weight: _____   Height: _____

Measurements: Chest: _____   Waist: _____   Hips: _____

　　　　　　Upper Arm: _____   Thigh: _____   Calf: _____

Sizes: Shirt _____   Pants: _____

Blood Pressure: _____

Resting Pulse Rate: _____

Number of sit-ups possible: _____

Number of push-ups possible: _____

How many flights of stairs can you climb before getting winded? _____

CHAPTER 6

The Big Three:

Cardio, Stretching and Weight Training

Activity is essential to staying active. It seems so simple and self-evident that everyone should realize it, right? Not necessarily. I don't think that anyone makes a conscious decision to be "inactive." It is simply something that creeps up on you, little by little until you realize you have to make some changes.

Maybe you weren't very active as a kid, maybe your family didn't engage in much physical recreation so you were never comfortable playing tennis or shooting hoops. Perhaps you always thought of yourself as uncoordinated so you have avoided aerobics classes, even though you would like to dance. It's not too late to find an activity that you enjoy! Experiment until you find something that feels right, or that is fun. Take a dance class. Rent a yoga video. Take a friend to the park to hit some tennis balls, or get a group to spend an evening bowling. Take advantage of technology and play the Wii. There are many sports and even entire workout programs available on the interactive system. It does not matter what activity you do you will still reap the benefits.

Many people think that because they walk the dog in the morning they don't need to work out. Wrong! You need to incorporate all three main types of exercise into your routine in order to reap the most rewards.

Exercise can be broken into several categories—cardio, stretching and weight training—and each has specific benefits for your body. Some activities, like swimming, span more than one category and are really great activities for conditioning, flexibility and strength training.

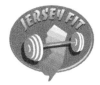

Cardio

Called aerobic exercise due to the way your body burns energy, it contrasts with strength training which burns energy anaerobically. What that means essentially, is that aerobic activities can be maintained for a longer time and help to burn stored fat. Aerobic exercise, or "cardio" as it is commonly referred to, has tremendous benefits for your body. Aerobic exercise is activity that increases your heart rate, pushing it to a level where it can gain efficiency. This level is called the target heart rate. Sources note that the target heart rate should be between 50 and 85% of your maximum heart rate, but that's hard to figure. One easy way is to determine your maximum heart rate is by subtracting your age from 220—your target zone should be 50 to 85 percent of that. For example, the target heart rate for a 50-year-old is 85-145 beats per minute. If you are still confused, the American Heart Association has an excellent page explaining target heart rate on their website (go to http://www.heart.org and search target heart rate). NOTE: If you have high blood pressure or take medication for high blood pressure, contact your doctor to determine your target heart rate.

The human body was designed to move, to be active, and much of that activity was intended to be aerobic. Programmed into your anatomy is something called the fight-or-flight response. When stressed—either by fear, anger or some other emotionally loaded situation such as frustration caused by unending demands—your body's primary reaction is to prepare to meet this challenge, whether that involves fighting off a foe or running from danger. Various hormones are released into your system which cause your heart to beat more rapidly, resulting in an increased heart rate, anxiety, sweating, a spike in blood sugar, and possibly shaking or twitching. The chemical changes in the body caused by activation of the fight-or-flight response are numerous and affect the function of nearly every bodily system—from interrupting digestion to subtly altering your vision. This complete, system-wide response is what makes chronic stress take such a huge toll on your health. The human body was designed to respond physically to a dangerous situation, not live full-time on "high alert."

A cardio workout can help you to burn off the chemical after-effects of daily stress. Many activities qualify as cardio, here are just a few:

Running - For ease and portability it is hard to beat running as an activity. Because it is a high impact exercise, it helps to strengthen your bones, and is superb at boosting your heart rate. If you start slow and build your endurance you can see excellent benefits from adding running to your routine.

Cycling - Indoors or out, cycling provides a great workout. You can easily regulate whether or not your heart is in the target zone depending on the intensity (speed and resistance) you are working at. It is considered a low impact workout, but use caution if you have knee issues. For a more structured workout try a spin class!

Swimming - Swimming is a marvelous activity for two reasons—it's low impact and it works your entire body. Water's natural buoyancy helps support your joints while providing resistance, making this an excellent choice for people who may be recovering from an injury. It is also a great activity for anyone who is afraid of falling. There are many water aerobics classes if you want to add a social aspect to your routine.

Walking - Although you only burn about half the calories walking instead of running, it is one of the easiest activities to incorporate into your life. You need a good pair of shoes—and that's about it! You can walk anywhere, indoors or out, so the weather is not a factor. The challenge with walking is to keep your heart rate in the target zone, but I highly recommend it as a simple exercise to get used to being active on a daily basis.

Skiing - Cold weather fans, this one's for you! Cross-country skiing is one of the top calorie burning activities around because it works both your upper and lower body. Of course, you can use the machine at the gym for the same benefits, but you lose out on the scenery!

Dance - Dance of all sorts provide good cardio benefits, but it also engages your mind due to the choreography, calms you because of the music, and has proven social benefits as well. Besides making you stronger and more flexible, recent studies are showing that dance can also cut the risk of dementia and may have an impact on Parkinson's as well.

Several machines at the gym can provide an excellent cardio workout. You can use the treadmill to walk or run, but there is also the elliptical trainer which offers a lower-impact workout, the stepper or stair climber, and the often overlooked rowing machine, which can give you a very intense full body workout.

If you want to enroll in a class, there's aerobics, step aerobics for a bit less impact (again, watch your knees on this one), kickboxing (fantastic upper and lower body workout), or the super popular calorie-burning Zumba. There are also a variety or yoga and Pilates classes, some of which are specifically geared towards keeping your heart rate in the target zone. If you would prefer to learn steps and movements in private, there are many videos and DVDs that will teach you any of the above and more in the comfort of your own home.

Your cardio workout should be fun! Go hiking with your family, grab a jump rope, do some body surfing at the beach, just get your heart rate up and keep it up! Start slow, build your endurance and you will be surprised at how quickly you can do more. Aim to do at least 20 minutes of cardio, three times a week.

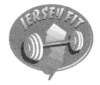

Stretching

Range of motion is a very important term, particularly as we age. The range of motion that you have in your joints can play an integral role in determining what activities you can do. Stretching is the way to increase your range of motion, and as such it is vitally important in helping you maintain productivity and independence.

The problem with stretching is that most people do it wrong. Forget what you learned in high school. Stretching a cold muscle is asking for injury—as is forcing or bouncing. If you apply the old adage "No pain; no gain" to your stretching, you will hurt yourself.

It may help to think of a muscle like a rubber band. Stretch a cold rubber band and it breaks. While your muscles or tendons may not actually break, they can tear, and your movement will certainly be affected during the healing process. You want to aim for a long, flexible, elastic muscle and you get that by stretching it. It is an excellent way to get blood flowing to a muscle that has been inactive—this is why the first thing dogs and cats do is stretch when they wake up.

Warm up for 10 or 15 minutes before stretching, or stretch at the end of your workout. Think slow, gentle, controlled movements with the goal of loosening and lengthening your muscles. You want to focus on each tendon or muscle group individually, hold a slow steady stretch for approximately 10 seconds and then switch to the other side.

If you have an injury or an area of particular concern, consult with your doctor or a physical therapist about the best way to stretch, and if possible have them guide you through the movement. Just because you are injured does not mean you should ignore that area! In fact, quite the opposite is true. Injured muscles and tendons can benefit greatly from the gentle movement of stretching, which helps maintain movement in the joint or tendon and boosts circulation and drainage.

Some of the exercises in the routine I give you incorporate stretching, but for a more in depth approach look into yoga. Yoga is an ancient practice that uses your own body weight as resistance and utilizes quite a lot of bending and stretching to increase flexibility, build muscle and calm the mind. Incorporating a few of the more basic stretch moves such as Downward Facing Dog, Warrior pose or Seated Twist pose can help you stay flexible.

Strength Training

Strength training is an anaerobic form of exercise focused on building muscle and increasing physical strength. As the name suggests, weight training is a type of strength training that uses weight machines or free weights to work your muscles. As a result, your muscles get stronger and larger.

Building muscle is important at any age, but the older you get, the more important it becomes. Weight training helps to reverse the loss of lean muscle mass that we have come to associate with getting older. Because muscle burns more calories than fat, even at rest, the more lean muscle you have the easier it will be to keep from packing on unwanted pounds. Weight training, by working the skeletal muscles, also helps keep your bones strong and can be a key component in staving off osteoporosis.

You do not need long workouts or enormous amounts of weight to see results. If you work each major muscle group twice a week, you will see results. You want to do 10-12 repetitions of each exercise, using a weight that is heavy enough to tire the muscles—in other words you want the last few repetitions to be difficult, but not so difficult that you cannot maintain proper form. As with aerobic exercise, start slow and gradually increase the amount of weight as your muscles get stronger. How will you know when it's time to up the amount of weight you are lifting? When the exercise becomes too easy.

Maintaining the proper form is essential. Use a controlled movement, both on the extension and the contraction. Allowing the weight to drop or swinging the weights to use the momentum to help you lift can result in injury. Lifting weights stresses the muscles—it can be very easy to extend too far or have a weight twist which can force the muscle or tendon out of or beyond its range of motion and possibly cause a tear or strain.

Most of the exercises that compose the routine in Chapter 9 utilize weights to help sculpt and define your muscles to make you slimmer and more toned and to make both your muscles and your bones stronger. To help avoid soreness and injury, I suggest you do each section—upper body, core, lower body—on successive days so that each group of muscles gets a day or two to rest. The process of strengthening a muscle involves making microscopic tears in the muscle fibers, and your body repairs these tears with new muscle fibers. The end result of the added muscle fiber is muscles that are bigger and stronger.

CHAPTER 7

Designing a Plan

Let's face it—life is a journey and without a well-designed plan it's like driving in circles all day long. When it comes to exercising and dieting the more detailed you are with your plan, the better your results will be. So what are some of the key factors to keep in mind when you are finally ready to design your exercise plan? Glad you asked.

You need to recognize that when you embark on this journey, you have to be willing to make a mental switch in order to accomplish your fitness goals. For most people, there is usually some event that serves as a wake-up call. But the catalyst is different for each person. For some people, it might be that they don't like the way they look anymore, or aren't happy with the size clothes they are wearing, or they are frustrated because they physically can't do what they used to do. For others, it may be a doctor's appointment or wellness visit and finding something of concern in test results or blood work results.

Your initial reaction, especially if it's to something the doctor has told you, may be fear. You may go into denial by blocking what they tell you but eventually you realize that you have to do something. At that point you're going to need some sort of plan or map for the rest of your journey.

A good place to start, if you haven't already, is with a visit to your doctor. Get a complete physical if it's been some time since you've had one. It's important to work with your doctor to establish your personal baselines, or starting points. This should include blood work, a blood pressure and heart rate check, and any other tests or lab work your practitioner may order for you.

After you've had a physical exam with your doctor and after you've gotten your doctor's recommendation, you can begin the process of designing and creating your plan of action. (For a list of questions to take to your doctor, see the Appendix at the end of this book.)

There are a number of areas that you need to take into consideration when you are designing a fitness plan for yourself. These include:

1. Your current physical condition.

2. Your goals and expectations.

3. Developing a balanced approach.

4. Setting a pace that works for you.

5. Choosing a plan you can stick to.

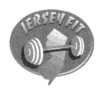

Change Is Up to You

It's no surprise that many people today are not satisfied with the way they look or how they feel. That would explain why the fitness industry, as a whole, has seen a tremendous growth in the last ten years alone. By the way, according to those experts, these projections are expected to continue to grow for many more years to come. Furthermore, as if we did not have enough to deal with, we are constantly reminded every day (whether through television, radio, print magazines or the internet) that our body image is becoming more relevant each and every day. So how do we go about analyzing what is right for us and our bodies? How should we best approach the right method and not let society dictate our goals?

Much like any other personal goals you may want to achieve, fitness goals must meet certain criteria in order for you to be successful. It's important for your fitness goals to be realistic, particularly if your goals include losing weight. You cannot expect to safely lose weight at a rapid pace. It is unrealistic to expect to lose more than one pound per week safely on any plan.

It's also important to have a method in place that allows you to measure your progress. You may want to go beyond tracking the number of pounds you lose. Maybe consider how much more energy you have, or track how much farther you can walk or run during your cardio workouts. It may be monitoring a health issue, such as blood pressure or cholesterol levels through your physician.

I've prepared a checklist of questions that you can ask yourself in order to set your own fitness goals and design a plan for yourself:

1) Do I want to improve my overall appearance or just focus on certain parts of my body?

2) Do I have any physical skills I want to improve or enhance?

3) Is my goal to build endurance, flexibility or strength or all three?

4) Is my goal strictly to lose weight?

5) Are my expectations realistic?

6) Do I want to make a lifestyle change?

7) Do I have a specific deadline for this goal?

8) Should I seek the services of a professional?

9) When was the last time I had a physical and is it time to go in for another one?

10) Am I mentally ready to make a change?

You can also choose to have a consultation with someone who can help you with your fitness program and set your goals. A professional, certified personal trainer will typically offer you a free consultation. From that initial meeting, the trainer will begin to get a sense of how to start helping you move forward with your fitness goals. And during your consultation, you can think about your fitness goals and really start to define them.

A trainer will likely start by reviewing goals with you—what's going on with your life, what made you consult a personal trainer in the first place. The trainer will want to know if you have something going on physically or medically that is making you want to start an exercise and fitness program. This could be tied to a number of reasons, or it could be the result of looking in the mirror.

In any case, your trainer will start out asking you a few basic questions, including:

Why are you consulting with a trainer?

What is it that is troubling you? Are you concerned about weight issues, health issues, strength issues, or a combination of things?

What goals are you trying to achieve?

Your trainer may also spend some time asking questions related to your general health and daily habits. For example, some of the questions I ask include:

What is your diet typically like?

How's your sleep? Are you getting enough sleep?

Are you taking medications and are you on a medication right now?

Some people find that their doctors can eliminate or lower the dosage on some medications once they start a regular exercise program.

A good personal trainer will be part of your personal health team. I am frequently in contact with some of the health care practitioners of my clients and sometimes work in conjunction with either a chiropractor or physical therapist.

In my own training practice, I have had consultations that have lasted an hour or longer just discussing goals. Part of the change in mindset has to be your realization that if you don't keep up with taking care of your body, your health will start to suffer. One of the key areas I reinforce with my clients is the necessity to make a mental change. The thought process required to change your life is going to take some work to become second nature. You have old habits and patterns to break and a new mindset to establish. Replace your old negative self-talk (*I can't believe I've let myself go so badly. I'm never going to get into shape. I hate to exercise.*) with positive messages (*I am taking charge of my health. I will be stronger next week. I can do this!*). As we saw in a previous chapter, your mind has a tremendous affect on your health, and even more on your ability to stay motivated.

The kids in school these days refer to negative self-talk as "self bullying." They are absolutely right in realizing that the mean things you say to yourself ARE damaging. Skeptical? Would you call the overweight woman in front of you at the bank "fat" to her face? If in a fit of sadness your child ate an entire bag of potato chips, would you berate him or her for having no willpower and tell them they are destined to be fat and miserable all their lives? If an elderly man at the doctor's office had difficulty climbing the stairs, would you mock him for being out of shape? The answer, of course, is no. Realize that you should be at least as nice to yourself as you are to strangers. Work on speaking to yourself in a supportive, friendly tone. When you make a mistake you are not an "idiot." You are human. And you are working steadily to make your life better.

Realize that the results are not going to be instantaneous. There's no such thing as quick fix. Programs that claim you will see rapid results do not work. There is always a current fad diet—it is usually ridiculously restrictive, maybe only letting you eat two or three things, and you would probably lose weight following it. But you will not be doing yourself any favors, and may actually be doing a great deal of harm to your body. And once you return to eating normally and living your life, any weight you lost will return, usually with a vengeance. People who starve themselves to drop a few quick pounds almost inevitably end up weighing more than when they started.

A balanced, sensible plan is the only way to lose weight and reclaim your health. So while it may take some time to see the results in the mirror, rest assured that with every workout tiny changes are taking place that will result in a stronger, healthier and shaplier you.

With that in mind, the sooner you start the sooner you will begin to see results.

CHAPTER 8

Before We Begin:

Some Exercise Basics

When learning any new skill, it is important to understand the fundamentals before beginning. It is only with a solid grasp of the basics that we can master any craft. Exercising is no different. In fact, the majority of people who do not learn proper form or technique run the risk of an injury... perhaps even a serious one. Before you start exercising there are a few things you should do:

Get clearance from your doctor. This is extremely important, especially if you have been sedentary or if you have health issues. The surest way to lose interest in fitness is to do too much at once—which can result in soreness or injury, or simply becoming overwhelmed and giving up. Tell your doctor that you are starting a fitness routine. Show him or her this book and discuss the changes you intend to make. Your doctor will be instrumental in helping to access where you are physically and pointing out any areas for modification.

Take all of your medications. Although in many cases people who make positive lifestyle changes can decrease some of their medications and possibly even discontinue them, that is a decision for you to make with your doctor. Allow me to repeat that. DO NOT reduce or eliminate any medications without consulting your doctor.

Think about whether or not you will want to hire a professional and gather as much information as you can. I have told you some things to look for when hiring someone to assist you in your lifestyle change, but nothing beats word-of-mouth referrals. Nobody is going to refer a trainer, a nutritionist, or any healthcare provider if they don't like them and if they didn't get results. Ask around—friends, associates, people in the fitness industry or those involved in sports or wellness such as health food or sports retailers, may be able to give you an informed opinion. If possible, ask for references.

Learn about fitness. Reading this book is an excellent first step, but if you are truly hoping to change your life and your future, you need to educate yourself. Read other exercise books, watch some exercise videos by reputable trainers. Be sure to check out my websites for instructional videos— www.TheRealFountainOfYouthBook.com or www.JerseyFitTV.com. You also can research more by logging on to the following sites:

The National Strength and Conditioning Association — www.nsca-lift.org

The American College of Sports Medicine — www.acsm.org

IDEA Health & Fitness Association — www.ideafit.com

An Internet search should yield many more informative websites, just be sure to check the credentials of the site and the people who post there. If someone advises something that seems odd, double-check with another professional.

Learning the way your body works is a key factor in the changes you are making. Having a grasp of how everything interacts makes it easier to institute changes that last, and every change, however minor, contributes to a healthier you. Something as simple as making sure that you bend your knees every time you lift a box will save wear and tear on your body, and keep it functioning better in the long run.

To understand how your body functions, it is important to distinguish the different muscle groups that make up the body. Here is a list of the major muscles and muscle groups:

Chest - composed primarily of the pectoral muscles, often referred to as pecs.

Shoulders - the main muscles here are the trapezius (which wrap over from the back) and the deltoids.

Back - several muscles make up the back area, the main ones being the trapezius (traps) at the top going over the shoulder and the latissimus dorsi (or lats) going from the armpit to the spine.

Arms - there are two major muscles that form the upper arm: the biceps in the front and the triceps in the back.

Front Thigh - the muscle at the front of the thigh is the quadriceps, often referred to as quads.

Back Thigh - the muscle at the back of the thigh is the hamstring.

Calves - the calf muscle is more properly called the gastrocnemius.

Abdominals - many muscles form your abdomen: the ones that run up the front of your abdomen and are responsible for the 6-pack appearance are called the rectus abdominis (or abs, for short); the muscles responsible for your waist on either side are the obliques.

Here is an illustration of the location of the above muscle groups:

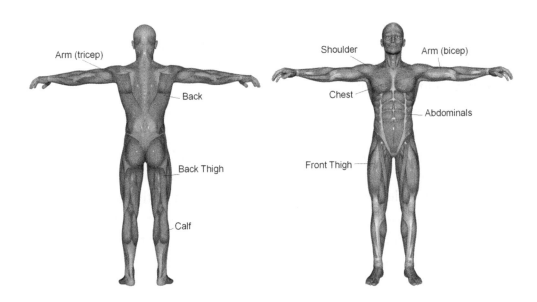

Before we go over the exercises I have chosen for you, it is extremely important to keep in mind a few pointers. These helpful tips will help you get ready to work out. I like to call these four P's of Preparation: Posture, Proficiency, Patience and Perseverance.

Posture: I am sure that all chiropractic professionals would agree with me that a proper stance is a key component to preventing injury. Try to keep your back straight or in a natural position when performing any exercise. If you feel any discomfort or unusual strain on your back you are most likely performing the exercise incorrectly. For example, when lying down on a bench always keep your head, shoulders, upper back, and lower back on the bench. Both of your feet should be flat on the ground as well.

Proficiency: To get the most out of your workout you will need to become adept at the exercises, and the best way to do that is to read each exercise all the way through, including any notes or modifications. Familiarize yourself with each step and study the photos for form.

Next, realize that in order to do each exercise properly, it is important to complete the full range of motion for each movement. In other words, whatever your starting position is where you will finish your exercise. The earlier you learn the proper technique the more proficient you will become and the faster you will make gains. Becoming proficient in the movements will also decrease the likelihood of injury.

Patience: They say that patience is a virtue and I couldn't agree more. Training requires time in order to see its results ... it cannot be done overnight. People who think they can achieve their goals in no time are sadly mistaken and will end up frustrated, disappointed, and quite possibly injured. Think about it— we are transforming your body, mind and soul. Rome was not built in a day, and your body shouldn't be either.

Perseverance: This is the key to your success. Nothing stands in your way. Every day is a challenge and only the strong willed can survive. Keeping those promises unleashes enormous energy and potential. All successful people have this trait, but don't despair if follow-through has been a problem for you. Perseverance can be learned, in fact, it is a habit you can cultivate. Start one day at a time and before you know it exercise will become a part your daily activity and perseverance will be a part of all that you do. That's what we want!

Keeping these qualities in mind—posture, proficiency, patience and perseverance—let's move on to the exercises. For those movements where posture is crucial, I will make a special note for you to focus on that. If, after reading through the instructions you are unclear on how an exercise should be performed, check my websites—www.TheRealFountainOfYouthBook.com or www.JerseyFitTV.com—where I have posted videos to demonstrate the proper form for many of the exercises included below. I will also highlight those exercises where you may need to have patience or which might require an extra degree of perseverance.

CHAPTER 9

The Exercises

Please Note: Breathing is very important when you exercise (and at all other times as well). You should always be exhaling air when exerting pressure, and inhaling at non-exerting pressure—in other words, once you are in position take a breath before you start the movement, exhale while you are performing the movement (lifting, pressing, squatting, etc.), and inhale again as you return to the starting position.

It is also helpful to tighten your abdominal muscles while performing the exertion phase of an exercise. Not only will this result in a better workout, it will help to increase stability.

Important!!

Once again, I need to stress that you should not begin this or any other exercise program without first checking with your doctor. Nothing in this book is intended to replace the advice of your healthcare provider.

Upper Body – **These exercises will target your chest, back, shoulders, biceps and triceps. Upper body work will make you stronger, enabling you to lift things more easily and will tighten and tone your arms.**

Dumbbell Bench Press

Start: Lie on your back on a bench with a dumbbell in each hand, one above each shoulder with palms facing out. Make sure your head, shoulders, and lower back are making contact with the bench and both feet are flat on the floor (this is called the five points of contact). Inhale.

Midpoint: Slowly press the weights straight up, exhaling as you go, until your elbows are fully extended.

Finish: Lower your weights to the starting position. Inhale and continue with your next repetition.

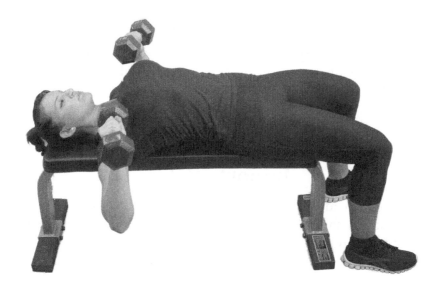

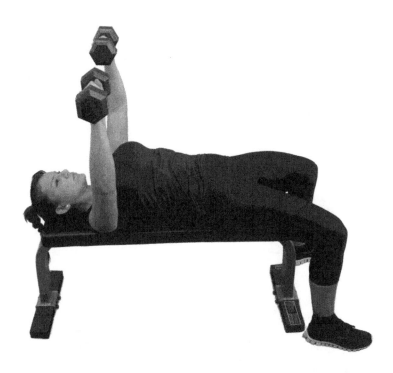

Notes: In this exercise it is important to concentrate on form. I suggest that men start with weights at 20-25 lbs, women should use 8-10 lbs to start. If you have trouble maintaining the proper form, use a lighter weight. This exercise will work your the muscles in your chest as well as your shoulders and your triceps.

Modifications: If you have shoulder or elbow problems, or problems with your lower back, do not perform this exercise. To make the exercises easier, raise one hand at a time instead of both at once. To increase the intensity, keep one hand straight up while you press with the other.

Dumbbell Bench Flies

Start and Finish: Lie on your back on a bench with a dumbbell in each hand and arms straight up with elbows fully extended and your palms facing in (don't forget about your five points of contact).

Midpoint: As you lower your weights (inhale a breath at the same time) you are basically doing a reverse hug. Bring the dumbbells out to the sides until your arms are parallel with the bench. DO NOT lower your arms beyond the parallel point as overextension may result in injury. Slowly raise the dumbbells to the starting position exhaling as you lift. Continue with your next repetition.

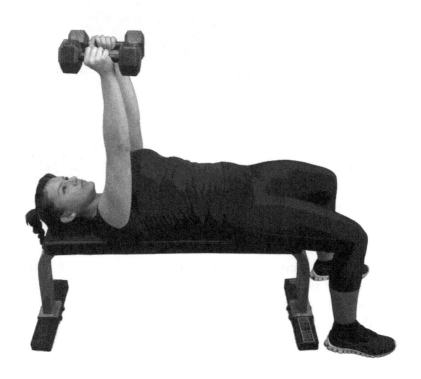

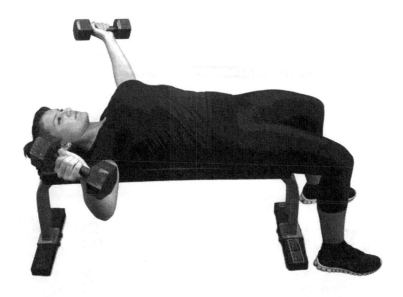

Notes: I recommend the same starting weight range as the Dumbbell Press. The previous exercise kept the weight centered over the body (called adduction); this one is a little harder (referred to as abduction) because the weight is being moved away from the body.

Modification: To modify, alternate your hands by holding one hand up straight while performing the movement with the other.

Seated Dumbbell Presses

Start and Finish: Sit on a bench with your back straight and both feet flat on the floor. Hold a pair of dumbbells in each hand, palms facing forward. Hold arms at shoulder height, elbows bent at a 90 degree angle.

Midpoint: Slowly press the dumbbells to full extension, keeping your back straight and your head looking forward. Slowly lower the dumbbells to the starting position and repeat.

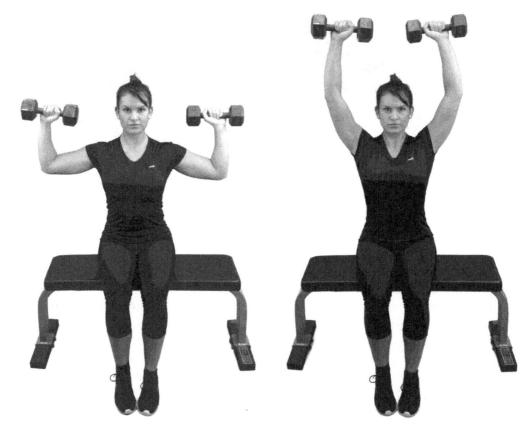

Notes: This exercise targets the shoulder area, but you need to be cautious about movements over your head, especially if you have an issue with your shoulders, because it does stress the area. It is very important to keep your back straight. Start with a comfortable weight. Do not to lean forward as it will throw off your form. Also, many people tend to move their hands forward as well as up. Be sure to go straight up, or you will not be able to maintain position.

Modifications: If you find that leaning forward is an issue because you need back support, you can sit in a chair. You can alternate hands as explained above, or you can change your grip on the dumbbells to palms facing in to make it easier.

Side Dumbbell Raises

Start and Finish: Stand upright with your feet shoulder with apart and your arms at your side. Hold a pair of dumbbells in each hand with palms facing in.

Midpoint: Keeping your arms straight, slowly lift the dumbbells until they are about level with your ears. Hold for a count of one and then slowly bring the weights down to starting position.

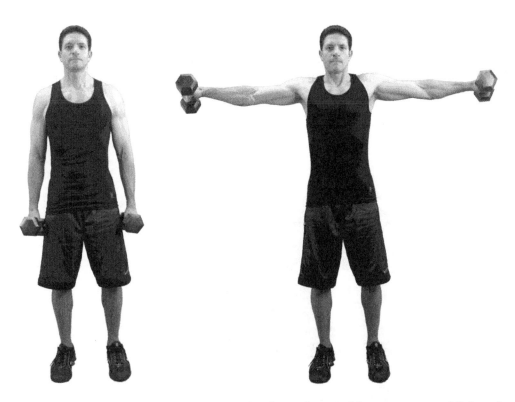

Note: Do not lean forward or backwards as this may put additional pressure on your back. I don't recommend using a belt as the powerlifters do, because it takes away support from the core and becomes a crutch. If you cannot lift the weights it means they are too heavy and you should use lighter weights to perform this exercise.

Modifications: This is a tough exercise because you are going against gravity. To make this movement easier, or if you find yourself having difficulty keeping your back straight, you can perform this exercise seated. To increase the difficulty, you can raise one hand at a time, or keep one hand up while working the other up and down.

One Arm Dumbbell Row

Start and Finish: To begin, place your right knee on the bench and your left foot flat on the ground. Lean forward until your back is parallel with the bench. Holding a dumbbell in your left hand, fully extend your arm so that it is straight down. Place your right hand on the bench, keeping your right arm fully extended as well. You should be looking straight ahead and your back should be nearly parallel to the floor.

Midpoint: Lift your left arm until your elbow is slightly above your back. Keep your back flat and your head looking straight ahead. Slowly lower the dumbbell and repeat. Apply the same principles for right side of your body.

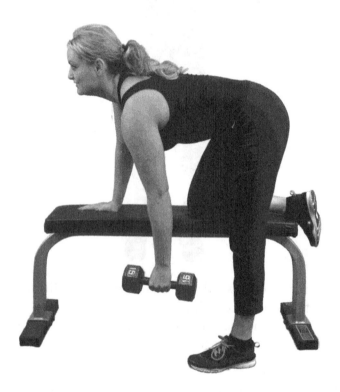

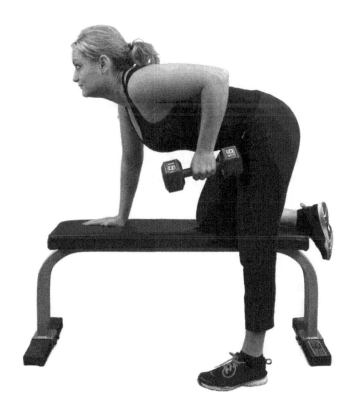

Note: This is an excellent exercise to build your lats (your back muscles), and it also works your biceps and shoulders. Most people use a bench for this, but you can also do this leaning forward to make more difficult, however it is important to keep the proper form so as not to put too much stress on the lower back. Make this exercise super hard by lifting one leg and holding it straight back throughout the movement.

Dumbbell Pullovers

Start and Finish: Lie across a flat bench with your shoulders and upper back resting on the bench. Keep your lower back slightly arched and both feet flat on the floor. Hold a dumbbell in each hand, palms facing forward. Raise the dumbbells overhead so that your arms are straight over your face.

Midpoint: Slowly lower your arms backwards until you reach a fully stretched position. Keep your shoulders on the bench and your lower back arched down with both feet on the ground. Return weights to start position and repeat.

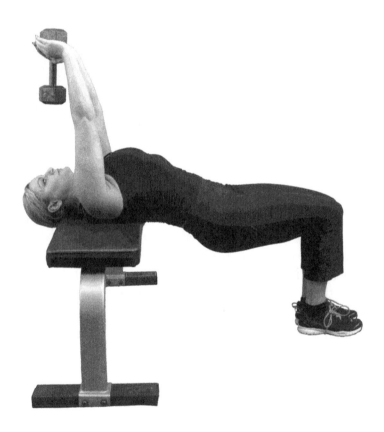

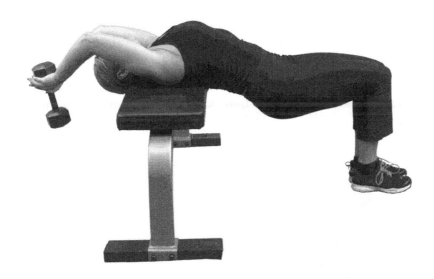

Note: Take care throughout this exercise as you are holding the weights over your face. Be sure that you have a firm grip on the dumbbells, and that your hands are not sweaty. In this movement, you are still working your back muscles when your arms go all the way back—but it is extremely important not to allow your arms to move beyond the line of parallel with your back. Doing so will result in overextension and can cause an injury.

Modifications: You can grip one dumbbell in each hand as written in the instructions, or you can hold one dumbbell with both hands as pictured above. This will make the exercise a little easier, and will give you a greater level of control. To securely hold a single dumbbell, spread both your hands. Overlap your thumbs and allow your index fingers to cross over each other, making a triangle space between your hands where the dumbbell will rest.

Bench Dips (Triceps)

Start and Finish: Start this exercise by standing next to a bench and turn so that your back is against it. Position your hands on the edge of the bench slightly more than shoulder with apart. Position your feet in front of you with the weight of body resting on your arms.

Midpoint: Lower your body slowly until your shoulders are parallel with your elbows—do not go past that point as it will place too much stress on your shoulders. Slowly straighten your arms to return to starting position.

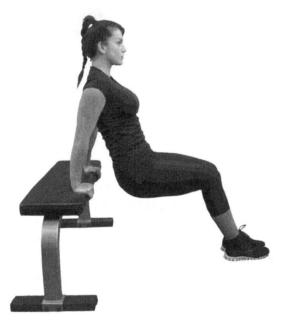

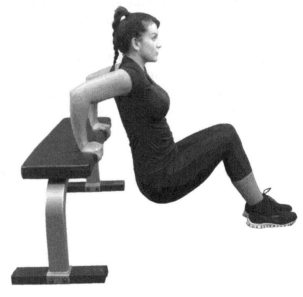

Notes: For the best tricep workout, stay as close to the bench as possible. The more you move away from the bench, the more your shoulders get involved. This is a tough exercise because you are using your body weight.

Modifications: If this movement is too difficult, please do not perform it. Another option is called a **triceps kickback**. To perform a triceps kickback, stand to the right of your weight bench, holding a dumbbell in your right hand, palm facing in. Bend your left leg and place your knee and lower leg on the bench; lean over and put your left hand on the bench as well. At this point, your body should be at a 45 degree angle.

To do the movement, bend your right elbow and move it back so that your upper arm is parallel to the floor. Keep your arm stable and close to your body and slowly kick back with your arm below the elbow, so that your entire arm is now parallel to the floor. Slowly lower the weight to the starting position and repeat. Turn around so that the bench is on your left, and switch the weight to your left hand. Place your right knee and hand on the bench, bend your left elbow and kick back with your left forearm.

Lying Bench Triceps Extension

Start and Finish: Lie down on a bench with a dumbbell in each hand, arms extended over your head palms facing in. Remember your five points of contact!

Midpoint: Bend your elbows and slowly lower the dumbbells toward your shoulder, not your head. Slowly raise the dumbbells to starting position.

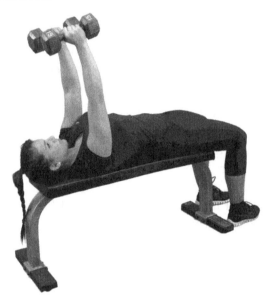

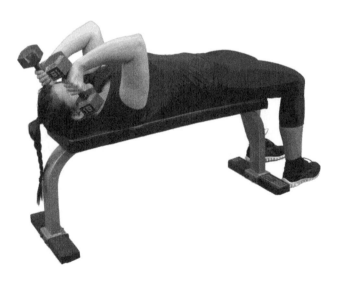

Seated Dumbbell Curls:

Start and Finish: Sit on the edge of a bench with your arms at your sides, dumbbells in your hands, palms facing forward.

Midpoint: Slowly lift the weights toward your shoulders, curling them up, until your palms are at chest level. Lower the weights to the starting point and repeat.

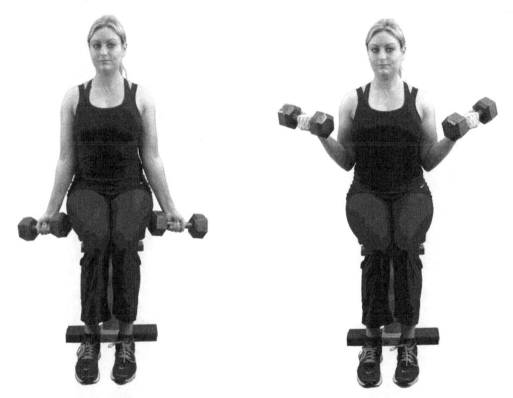

Notes: This exercise is designed to target your biceps (lower arms). Be cautious if you have elbow or lower back problems. As with the previous exercises, if you find yourself leaning forward you may use a chair instead of a weight bench for support.

Hammer Curls:

Start and Finish: Stand straight with dumbbells down at your side (palms facing each other) and feet shoulder with apart.

Midpoint: Slowly raise dumbbells (keeping palms facing each other) until they reach the top of your shoulder. Keep your back straight, do not lean forward or back.

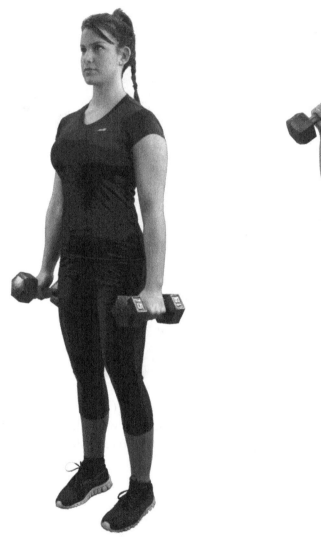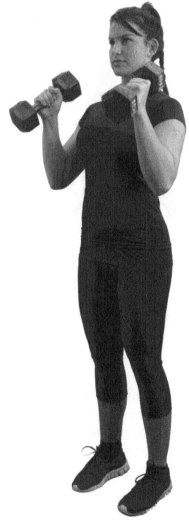

Note: This exercise focuses mainly on your biceps. Do not lock your knees, as this will tend to throw off your posture, and place strain on your lower back.

Lower Body – These exercises will target your legs, especially your gluteus, quadriceps, hamstrings and calves.

Dumbbell Squats:

Start and Finish: Hold two dumbbells by your side with your palms facing in. Stand with your back straight and your feet shoulder width apart.

Midpoint: Slowly lower your body while keeping your back straight, shoulders back and your head looking forward. Make sure you do not let your knees go past your toes. Hold for a count of one and raise your body to starting position.

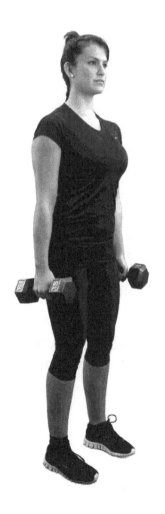
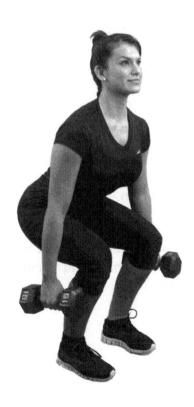

Notes: This exercise works your butt and your hamstrings, but mainly it targets your quads. If you have hip, knee or lower back problems, you should limit the range of motion with this exercise, moving only a few inches at first until you see how much strain this places on your joints.

Modifications: To make this exercise easier, eliminate the dumbbells, or use a stability ball on your back against a wall. Usually your legs are shoulder width apart, some people find widening your legs helps, or use a bench—squat until you feel the bench and then come back up. It is recommended to only go parallel to floor with your legs; farther than that can cause too much strain on the joints. To make this exercise more challenging, once you master the form try holding the dumbbells by your side, straight overhead or holding them straight out to engage your shoulders as well.

Dumbbell Lunges:

Start and Finish: Hold two dumbbells by your side with palms facing in. Toes should be pointed forward, your back straight, shoulders squared and head looking forward.

Midpoint: Step forward with your right foot. Bend at your knees and lower your body until your back knee is a few inches above the floor. Make sure your front knee does not extend past your toe and is pointed in the same direction as your knee. Push back with your right leg to return to the starting position. Repeat the same movement with your left leg.

Notes: Perfect the squat before you move on to this exercise. As in the squat, proper form and technique must be followed to prevent injury, particularly to the knee.

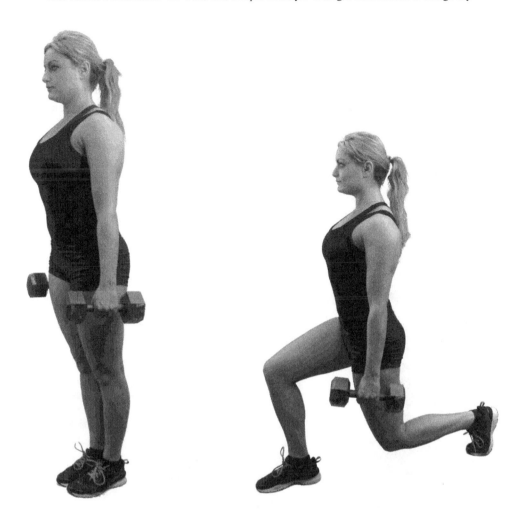

Modifications: To decrease the intensity of this exercise eliminate the dumbbells. There is a lot of core interaction in this movement, and it puts more stress on your forward knee, so start off without dumbbells and be really careful not to over-extend (move your knee in front of your toes) especially if you have knee issues. To make this exercise harder, hold the dumbbells overhead or use a kettle bell. My favorite variation is to hold the kettle bell straight up. You can add elevation, step up onto a step in a lunge or even more intense would be to start on the step and step down into your lunge. There are bonus points if you step backwards! Side lunges are good as well to vary the routine and to work slightly different muscles.

Straight-Leg Deadlifts:

Start and Finish: Stand straight while holding dumbbells in front of you with palms facing toward your legs. Shoulders should be back, head forward and feet shoulder width apart.

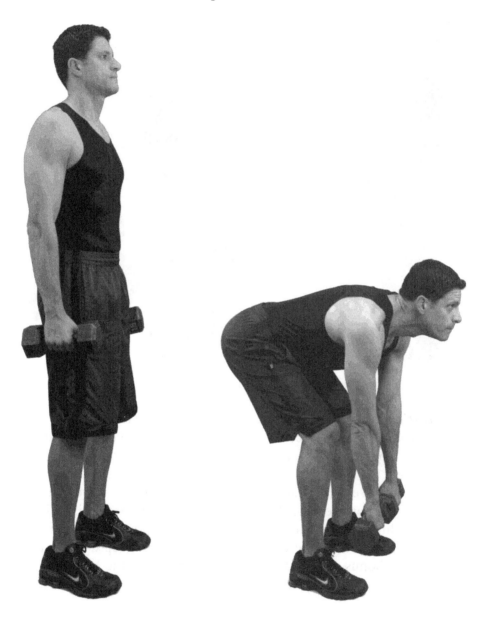

Midpoint: Slowly bend your body forward at the hips and lower the dumbbells until they almost touch the floor. Keep your back straight throughout the exercise. Your head should look forward. Hold for a count of one and slowly raise your upper body to starting position.

Notes: If you have some back issues, be careful with this exercise. Be sure to keep your back as straight as possible as this exercise is to focus on the hamstrings, not on using your back muscles to lift with.

Modifications: To make this movement easier simply eliminate the weights. For a harder workout, increase the weights or use a barbell.

Calf Raises:

Start and Finish: Stand straight with dumbbells at your side held with your palms facing in toward your legs. Your feet should be shoulder width apart with your toes facing outward.

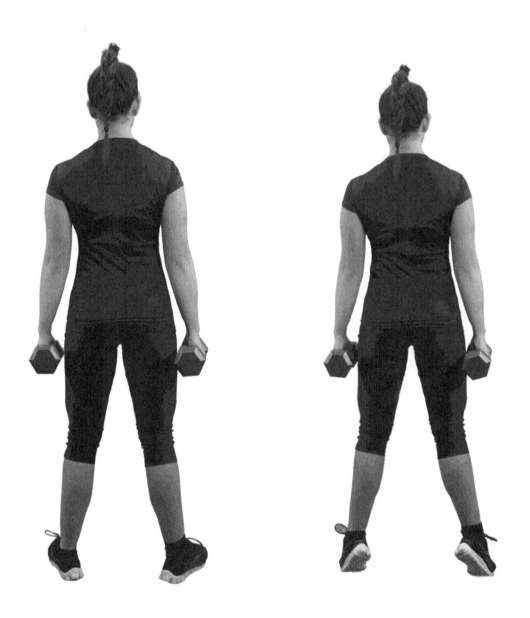

Midpoint: Slowly raise your heels until you reach full extension. Hold for a count of one and lower your feet to starting position.

Notes: These are simple, you can do them anywhere - you use your own body weight. These are a good thing to do while you are waiting in line at the grocery store. Calf raises obviously work your calves, but the focus is on the muscle that defines the size and shape of your calves.

Modifications: The easiest way to perform this exercise is to stand on a flat floor as shown, you can't get full range of motion, but you can get a burn. To increase the intensity and to work the entire calf muscle, do this movement on an aerobic step or on stairs, and allow your heels to drop below the stair as you come down. For an even harder workout add weights. Walk on your toes like a ballerina!

Hip Front/Back (with ankle weights):

Start and Finish: Strap an ankle weight to your left ankle and stand straight up. Keep your hands at your waist and look forward.

Midpoint: Slowly raise your left leg in front of you until it is parallel with the floor. After a count of one, return the leg to starting position. Slowly raise your left leg behind you until maximum stretch is achieved and hold that position for a count of one. Lower your leg to starting position and repeat. Switch the ankle weight to your right leg and repeat the process.

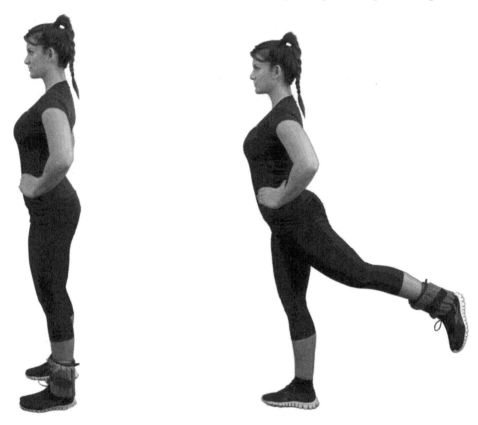

Notes: This is a great exercise. A lot of my clients call this a killer, but it will strengthen your hips, which is why this is such a beneficial exercise for older people. Be sure to stand up tall throughout this exercise—engaging the muscles in your core to keep your balance is part of what makes this movement so effective. I suggest that you start this exercise without weights to make sure you have the form and the movement down, and then add weight as you increase in proficiency.

Modifications: To make this exercise easier, use a chair or put your hand on a wall, and use that to help yourself balance. Again, think ballerina. To increase the difficulty of this movement, do not use anything for support, and add the ankle weights.

Hip Side (with ankle weights):

Start and Finish: The starting position for this exercise is the same as for the Hip Front / Back. Strap an ankle weight to your right ankle and stand straight up. Keep your hands at your waist and look forward.

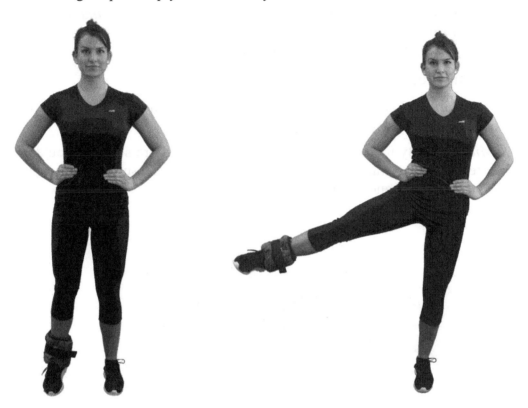

Midpoint: Slowly raise your right leg out to your side as far as you can (your ultimate goal is to have your leg parallel to the floor). Hold for a count of one then lower your leg to the starting position. Perform all repetitions, then switch the ankle weight to left leg and repeat process.

Notes: Your pelvic girdle (the group of bones that provides support for the trunk and to which the muscles that move your legs attach) is extremely important. There have been studies which show they can determine how long you will live after you break your hip, and although the timeframe varies, depending how active you were, your weight, etc. current reports indicate that roughly one quarter of people 65 and over who break their hip die within the year, and one-half are unable to return to their former physical capabilities.

Modifications: The modifications for this exercise are the same changes as above. To make this exercise easier, put a hand on a chair or the wall for support. To make this movement more difficult, do not use anything for balance and add the ankle weights, as described.

Core Exercises – **Your core consists of the abdominal muscles, the obliques and the muscles in the back. This group of exercises will help strengthen your waist. A strong core is essential for balance.**

Note: When performing core exercises it is extremely important to maintain proper form. No pressure should be placed on the back of your head or spine. Please follow directions carefully.

Floor Crunches:

Start and Finish: Lie face up on the floor with your hands beside your ears, knees together and feet flat on floor.

Midpoint: By focusing on your midsection, slowly raise your shoulders just a few inches upward being careful not to put any pressure on your neck. Hold for a count of one and return to start position.

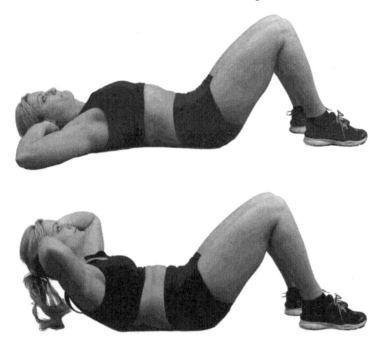

Notes: This is as basic as it gets. You DON'T need to rise very far from the floor, just a few inches, but be sure your form is right so you don't stress your neck.

Modifications: To make this exercise harder, put your feet on a chair or use a dumbbell over your head. For even more core engagement, instead of lying on the floor, use a stability ball. To make it even harder increase the elevation. The hardest of all is to do this exercise inverted or hanging. For those who can't get on the floor, you can do these on a bed.

Sit Ups:

Start and Finish: As with the crunches above, to start this exercise lie face up on the floor with your arms straight and beside your body. Your legs should be bent, with feet slightly apart and flat on the floor.

Midpoint: Slowly raise your torso to a sitting position by keeping your head in a fixed position and arms straight out in front of you. Keep your feet flat on the ground. Hold for a count of one and return to start position.

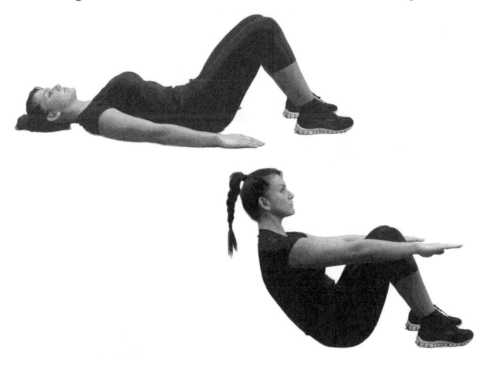

Note: This exercise differs from the Crunch in that you actually bring your whole torso up. You can vary the hand position in this exercise to find what's most comfortable. You can extend your arms and hold them out straight as shown, you can place your hands by your ears as shown in the photo for the Crunch, or you can cross your arms over your chest and perform the sit-up that way. So long as you DO NOT place your hands behind your head and use them to help pull yourself up, you can use any of those arm positions that you prefer.

Modifications: To make this movement easier, stick your feet under the couch or have someone hold them. Difficulty can be increased by performing sit ups on a stability ball, a decline bench, by adding weights, or by doing this inverted.

Bent Knee Leg Raises:

Start and Finish: Lie face up on the floor with your hands beside your body and under your buttocks. Fully extend your legs and keep your feet together. Your head should be resting on the floor.

Midpoint: Raise your feet off the ground and bring your knees toward your chest to form a 90 degrees angle or greater. Lower your legs slowly, being sure to keep them under control and not letting your heels touch the floor. When you are approximately 1 inch from the ground immediately raise your legs back up for the next repetition.

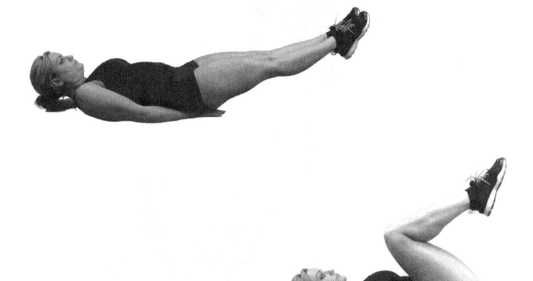

Notes: For support, keep your hands underneath your tush (glutes) as shown above. If you are looking for variety, alternate your legs, doing first one then the other.

Modifications: For an easier movement, start with your feet on the floor and your knees already bent. To make it harder, fully extend your legs and continuously keep them off the floor, and then bring to your chest. To up the intensity further, you can use ankle weights.

Planks:

Start and Finish: Begin by getting into a pushup position. Your legs should be extended back with balls of your feet on floor. Bend your elbows and rest your weight on your forearms.

Midpoint: Brace your core and hold this position for as long as possible. Each time you perform this exercise, try to hold it a little longer.

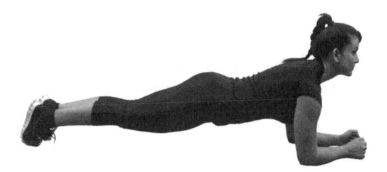

Note: I love Planks—they are the best core exercise. Yes, it can be difficult, but proficiency is just a matter of practice. As I explained in the Fitness Assessment section, the Plank is an excellent indicator of your core strength.

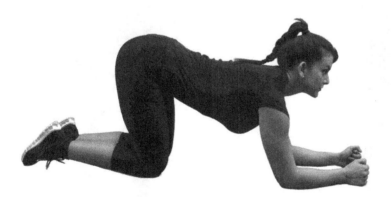

Modification: Make the Plank easier by starting on your knees, but be sure to use a mat or cushion as this may hurt your knees. For a harder Plank, lift one arm, like a tripod. Raise intensity also by going on an incline, or use a bench, balancing with your forearms on the bench. The key here is the duration.

Side Bends:

Start and Finish: Stand upright with your back straight and your head looking forward. Hold a dumbbell in each hand with palms facing your legs.

Midpoint: Bend from your waist to the right side, while sliding your right arm down your right leg. Slide your right hand up your leg in a controlled motion to straighten and return to the original position. Repeat on the left for a count of one. Be sure to return to the starting (upright) position in between!

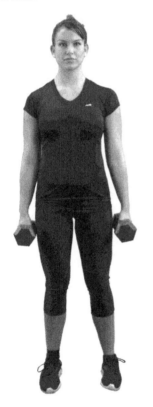 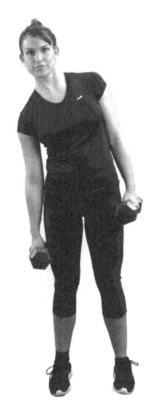

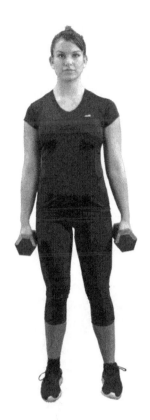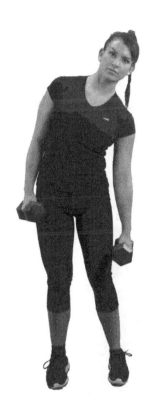

Notes: Side bends target your oblique muscles which will help define your waist. The goal here is to perform these exercises in a smooth controlled movement, so that you feel a pull each time as you gently stretch the muscles. NO bouncing, as that can result in injury!

Side Twists (w/medicine ball):

Start and Finish: Stand upright with your feet shoulder width apart and your head looking forward. Hold a medicine ball at chest level with both arms extended.

Midpoint: Slowly rotate your torso to your right while keeping arms, head and medicine ball in front of you. Hold for a count of one. Rotate your torso back to starting position, again holding for a count of one. Slowly rotate your torso to your left while keeping everything the same. Hold for a count of one and then return to starting position.

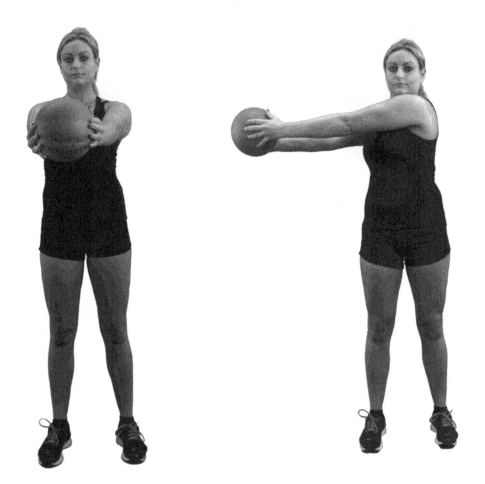

Note: This is another excellent exercise for building strength and flexibility in your core and adding definition to your waist.

Modifications: Vary the intensity of this exercise by adjusting the amount of weight you use. Remember this is a stretch, so you want to feel a gentle pull in the muscle.

CHAPTER 10

Nutrition is Essential

As I said earlier, productive longevity is a complex issue, and will need more than just exercise to attain. Integral to getting healthier and feeling better is revamping the way you eat. The old adage that you are what you eat is true. Unfortunately, too many people are unaware of what they are actually putting in their mouths.

Once upon a time just about everyone ate food fresh from the garden. There are many reasons for this shift, but despite the ease and convenience of pre-packaged, processed food, the nutritional value of a box of fruit snacks is not the same as an actual, fresh apple. Once you start eating fresh, whole food, I guarantee you will feel a difference.

To help you understand how proper nutrition can change the way you look and feel, I have interviewed Dr. Lori Magoulas. Dr. Magoulas is a registered dietitian with a PhD in Molecular Nutrition and a Master of Science from the Institute of Human Nutrition at Columbia University, New York, with a concentration in molecular nutrition, body composition and resting metabolic rate.

She has both clinical and research experience as a dietitian and has been in private practice as a medical nutrition therapist since 1996. Her scientific research included basic science research in the nutrient regulation of gene expression in a laboratory that focused on heart disease and its causative factors.

She is currently in private practice in Monmouth County, New Jersey.

I spoke with Dr. Magoulas about her background in nutrition. She also discussed with me the role of nutrition in productive longevity and how the proper nutrients can be part of an overall fitness regime.

How is your educational and professional background unique compared with many dietitians?

My background is unique in that there are generally not many dietitians with a PhD, with both basic science research and clinical practice experience. One of my goals is to translate the science behind nutrition and disease research in a way that the layperson can easily understand, as well as to promote behavior change that is lasting.

I've worked with patients of all ages, from pediatrics to geriatrics, in private practice, in a hospital setting and in nursing homes. I've also had long standing affiliations with the American Cancer Society, the American Diabetes Foundation and the Academy of Nutrition and Dietetics. In my affiliation with the American Cancer Society I've developed and presented programs discussing the role of nutrition and exercise in cancer prevention.

Why did you decide to study nutrition?

Since high school, I have had a strong interest in both science and in working with people, so I looked for a way to combine those interests. Human nutrition became the focus of my studies as an undergraduate student at Cook College, Rutgers University.

Can you explain how nutrition can affect longevity?

Nutrition can affect longevity because what we eat can have both direct and indirect effects on how the body functions. Through these effects, longevity can be altered.

The basic nutrients that make up a person's diet—macronutrients, micronutrients and phytonutrients— all play a role in longevity. Macronutrients—which include proteins, fats and carbohydrates—provide fuel, promote tissue maintenance and repair as well as build muscle. Micronutrients, or vitamins and minerals, act as the building blocks for hormones and enzymes. Phytonutrients, which are nutrients from plants, can aid the body in fighting disease and also help the body with optimal functioning.

Productive longevity is a state where the body functions optimally while keeping disease at bay. This will allow quality of life to be improved. There are processes that go on as a normal function of aging, and there are effects on the body from long-term exposure to chemicals and the environment. Along with natural cellular aging that affects everyone, there are environmental factors affecting the body, such as responses to pollution, chemicals, breaking down prescription drugs. Once these chemicals are inside the body, they put an extra burden on your system. However, proper nutrition can possibly buffer or balance these environmental insults and protect the body as it ages.

What do we need from the nutrients in our diet?

Our diet provides important things that our body uses to do what it does on a daily basis. The food we eat provides many nutrients as substrates or co-factors to many of the chemical processes that occur daily in the body as part of normal functioning. The better we eat, the better our body functions, like a well-oiled machine. Vitamins and some minerals plug into the chemical pathways of the body and can therefore play a role in optimal functioning.

However, equally important is that deficiencies in the diet may also have an effect on longevity. For example, overnutrition, or eating too much, can lead to factors such as elevated body weight. There are studies indicating that elevated body weight can be linked to an increases in generalized inflammation, or what is also known as silent inflammation, an underlying premise of conditions including heart disease.

Conversely, undernutrition, which includes not eating enough or having a diet that is deficient in nutrients, can impair the body's ability to maintain optimal health and functioning, and can lead to disease. Undernutrition can be defined in a number of ways and includes not taking in enough nutrients, or not having enough of a variety of macro and micronutrients, or not eating the right way to get enough vitamins and minerals for the body to function properly. A lack of protein in the diet of the older population can also be linked to a lot of issues, such as decreased muscle mass.

Why is nutrition such an important part of a fitness regime?

We know that the largest decline in muscle mass is seen in people over the age of 60.

Nutrients are an important component of any fitness regime because they provide energy and because they are the building blocks for muscle formation and repair. Proper nutrition and dietary intake allow the best results to be achieved from exercise and strength training.

Exercise can have both physical effects and metabolic effects. When people exercise they are commonly looking to improve their health in a variety of ways. For example, they may be looking to lose or gain weight, gain strength and muscle mass, improve their fitness level, resculpt their body, or improve cholesterol, blood pressure or even blood sugar levels.

However, you may not experience the full result of what you are trying to achieve if you don't have the proper nutrition to go along with it. For example, if you over-consume calories, you will be more likely to put on weight, which could cancel the calorie-burning effect of the cardio exercises you engage in.

Exercise itself, as well as normal bodily functioning, creates a metabolic stress on the body in the form of free radicals. Proper nutrition can help the body better deal with those byproducts.

Can you give us a starting point for beginning an optimal healthy diet?

Certainly, there are some basics that anyone can implement right away:

- Don't skip meals.
- Include each of the food groups in your diet every day.
- Eat at least three meals a day. Try to balance them.
- Phase out sugar-sweetened beverages.
- Omit deep-fried foods.
- Do not over-consume animal fats.

What are some specific food choices people can make to promote longevity and create a balanced diet?

Fruits and Vegetables: For starters, fruits and vegetables are the foundation of a diet to promote longevity because of all the fabulous phytonutrients (nutrients found in plants) and the abundant vitamins that they contain. The easiest way to make sure you're getting enough fruits and vegetables, and the right ones, is to include them in your meals several times a day. Choose a variety of colors and aim for five or more servings per day.

Lean Proteins: Also a must. There is a problem with the aging population getting enough protein in their diet. Adequate protein is necessary to prevent loss of muscle mass. Lean choices include chicken, fish, lean beef, turkey, egg whites and low fat cheeses.

Healthy fats: It is very important not to eliminate all fats from your diet. Fat provides many benefits, and the Omega 3 and other healthy fats are necessary for a number of reasons, including helping to decrease inflammation in the body. Many adults do not get enough Omega 3 fatty acids in their diet. Some good sources of Omega 3's include cold water fish, flaxseed oil, chia seeds and walnuts. Other good choices for oils include nuts, seeds, olive and canola oils.

Other necessary nutrients: Vitamin D needs to be added to the diet in the form of a supplement, along with Calcium and Magnesium. It's also important to include calcium-rich foods such as lowfat milk, yogurt and cheeses in your diet. Other good calcium sources include spinach and kale. I also recommend a good multi-vitamin (without iron—men and menopausal women do not need the extra iron). Vitamin D is necessary for the body to absorb calcium.

Can you discuss some age-related issues that are related to proper nutrition?

There are a number of common age-related issues that are tied to nutrition and diet, including the following:

Loss of muscle mass: This can be a cause of a variety of problems in the aging population. The loss of muscle mass often begins around the age of 60, and can lead to various physical limitations, including decreased balance, speed and agility. A proper diet and especially adequate protein intake can help boost muscle mass.

Bone Loss: This is an issue in both men and women that can also lead to physical limitations and increases the risk of fractures. Including calcium and Vitamin D in your diet can help combat bone loss.

Chewing issues: In the elderly and even other populations, chewing issues can have a drastic affect on diet and nutrition because these issues can alter their eating habits by limiting the types of foods they eat and by interfering with the proper breakdown of food.

Lack of skills or interest in cooking: An inability or a lack of interest in preparing meals can especially be a problem with older people who live alone, such as widows, widowers, or even empty-nesters who no longer have to cook for a big family. They may tend to not have the best diet and overly rely on processed or prepared foods that have high sodium contents.

Sleep changes: Poor sleep is common in the older population, who often suffer from insomnia and interrupted sleep patterns.

Economics: Because of their fixed incomes, some elderly people simply can't afford to buy high quality food, especially high quality fresh fruits and vegetables. Part of the role of the health community is to educate and convince people that it is necessary to eat healthy and that it must be part of their monthly budget.

Medications: Both prescription and non-prescription medication can affect how your body absorbs nutrients, or can affect the appetite.

What tips can you give to help people stay on track and focused on maintaining good nutrition?

For starters, you need a way to begin weaving nutrition into your game plan. You can accomplish this in a number of ways. For example, you can implement the same meal plan week after week and then this weekly plan can dictate your shopping list. Or, if you prefer, you can shop more often and decide what you are going to eat on a daily basis. However, planning ahead of time will make is easier to accomplish your nutrition goals.

One thing that can help with meal planning is to realize that good, nutritious meals can be a fusion of pre-prepped foods (such as vegetables that have been cut for use in a variety of dishes and recipes) and foods prepared from scratch. Dinner can be a combination of leftovers, or some leftovers plus one thing cooked that night.

For example, you can start by grilling a large batch of boneless, skinless chicken breasts. Use some for dinner one night, slice some up with salad for lunch the next day, and add them to a vegetable stir-fry on another day. You can cook extra rice or other grains and vegetables so that you can use them as side dishes for more than one night, or even as a lunch.

Using your imagination and being inventive with possibilities can liberate you and allow you to enjoy putting meals together. Planning in this way can eliminate having to cook from scratch every single day if you don't want to.

Some people feel that following a diet may be too restrictive and they become concerned that they will be deprived of certain foods. Can you address this issue?

Everyone needs to determine how much of a role unhealthy foods play in their overall dietary intake. I would tell someone that in order to do this, you need to take an honest look at your eating habits by keeping a food journal of exactly what you eat for a few days or a week. Then look at your results from a dietary perspective and try to identify your patterns and habits. This food journal should include what you eat, the amount you eat, even the time of day you eat. You can then see what you have too much of or not enough of. Sometimes you'll find that the unhealthy foods crowd out the healthy ones. You need to begin by finding a balance.

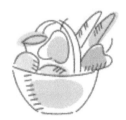

CHAPTER 11

Framework

When training my clients, I consider myself to be a part of their personal health team. I sometimes work in conjunction with my personal training clients' doctors, physical therapists or other health practitioners. Very often, clients contact me because their physician has recommended that they start a fitness program to achieve any number of health goals. Even if they're contacted me for other reasons, I always begin every consultation with an assessment of my new client's current physical condition as it's essential for a personal trainer to be aware of any medical issues that their client may have, as well as any medication they are taking.

I feel very strongly about the benefits of chiropractic care and it is an integral component of my personal wellness program. I schedule regular visits with my chiropractor so he can constantly evaluate my spinal alignment as it is crucial for staying fit.

I am very fortunate to have been able to interview two local experts in the field of chiropractic medicine for this book. Dr. Larry Arbeitman and Dr. Sharon Barnum are licensed chiropractors in New Jersey and have agreed to provide some excellent information on how chiropractic care can complement your fitness program and fitness journey, and how spinal alignment can bolster productive longevity.

A Conversation with Dr. Larry S. Arbeitman

Dr. Larry S. Arbeitman is a Magna Cum Laude graduate of Logan College of Chiropractic, St. Louis, Mo. An upper cervical practitioner, he is in private practice in Monmouth County, New Jersey.

Please tell us about your background and what attracted you to the field of chiropractic medicine.

I've been a practicing chiropractor since 2003. What attracted me to the field of chiropractic medicine was the fact that people got well by facilitating the body's natural healing properties. It's the largest non-drug healing area.

Can you elaborate on the type of care that you provide?

Chiropractic care is so much more than just back and neck pain. I specialize in upper cervical care. There are fewer than 2000 upper cervical practitioners worldwide and they comprise less than 1% of chiropractors in the U.S.

Upper cervical practitioners work with the central nervous system. What I do involves gentle, specific adjustments to the upper cervical spine to remove misalignments called vertebral subluxations.

The central nervous system (CNS) controls the entire body and poor lifestyle choices can severely negatively affect the central nervous system. Chiropractic adjustment allows the entire central nervous system to operate at a higher level. The structure of the body determines how well the body works. A healthy central nervous system is absolutely necessary for the body to be well. Because the CNS drives the heart and lungs, it is of vital importance that the CNS be healthy and aligned.

How can chiropractic care be part of a fitness program?

The wellness chiropractor helps patients by educating them and giving strategies. People can incorporate chiropractic care as part of an overall health and wellness strategy.

Athletes know that alignment is an integral part of a fitness program. Exercising on a crooked framework can be good for your heart and lungs but terrible for your joints. This is why many injuries occur while people are working out.

What kind of exercise should you be doing with a spinal condition?

If someone has a spinal condition, research shows that they need to get moving – exercise is a necessity. However modifications may need to be made to their exercise program, or they may possibly require an exercise regime custom tailored for their condition. The bottom line is that you don't want to stop moving because you have a spinal problem. You need to find out what you should be doing despite the condition.

How can chiropractic care help promote longevity?

What's happening to much of our population and society and our health is largely related to stress.

We are being subjected to more stress than ever before. I see this in heart rate variability – this is the gold standard when it comes to measuring stress and can indicate that the body has moved into fight or flight mode which is the body's natural response to stress or danger. What happens is that when the body's flight or fight response is triggered it shunts blood away from the stomach, causing you to lose your appetite. Because the body needs energy (supposedly to run away or to fight) it dumps sugar and cholesterol into your bloodstream. This surge in glucose and cholesterol stresses the immune system. This in turn results in an increased heart rate, blood pressure and spikes in blood sugar levels.

What I am finding in my practice is that the majority of people are running in chronic fight or flight mode, which means they are constantly on alert—their body is under stress 24 hours a day. Their adrenal glands become completely burned out because of running under stress all of the time. Many people counter this by living on energy drinks and caffeine to gain energy.

We may not be able to get rid of all of the stress of modern life but we do need to have strategies. Chiropractic adjustment should be one of those strategies. It is the safest way to shut off the fight or flight mode.

What do you think is one of the main contributors to productive longevity?

Probably the main thing – people need to have a purpose greater than themselves. Studies show that people living past 100 have a great sense of purpose and an optimistic, positive outlook. Some lifestyle choices can determine how well your golden years will be. Chronological age and biological age are two very different things.

Also, optimism and ambition both affect longevity. People who look on the bright side often live longer than those who don't really try to be happy.

What would you consider to be one of the most challenging aspects of attaining fitness?

There are psychological reasons why people don't make changes – they become overwhelmed, uncertain and basically end up paralyzed about making that decision.

One of the best things you can do for yourself is find a person or expert who can guide you so that you don't have to go it alone. It may be a personal trainer, or a nutrition counselor – it's important to find the right quarterback who can help you plan it out.

After finding that guide, the next step should be to change just one thing so that you can get started and then stick with that change. Be careful not to do too much at first. But take that one thing – that one change – and make it a habit. Then add other things, also one at a time.

The other important thing to note when you have made the decision to get fit is to realize that it's never too late and don't give up. Even if you're 70 years old, take an action every day to keep moving forward to health.

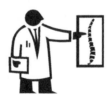

A Conversation with Dr. Sharon Barnum

Dr. Sharon L. Barnum is a graduate of Kean University and Los Angeles College of Chiropractic. In private practice since 1991, she is the owner of A and A Chiropractic in Monmouth County, New Jersey.

Can you describe your background?

I have a Bachelor's degree in Biology and then studied at Los Angeles College of Chiropractic. I also take continuing education credits and keep up to date with pain management developments.

I've been in private practice since 1991, at first in Pennsylvania and then in New Jersey. I'm currently practicing in Monmouth County, New Jersey.

I am a neuromusculoskeletal practitioner. I normally see patients who are in pain or who have some sort of disability. Chiropractors and physical therapists often treat the same sort of patients. However, chiropractic care is not only about aches and pains. While patients may begin seeing a chiropractor because of pain or an issue, over the long term, many patients also see there are many other benefits to being adjusted regularly.

Can you provide some examples of some of these benefits?

For example, elderly patients who see a chiropractor regularly tend to have fewer falls and hospitalizations than those who don't. Studies also show that people who get adjusted regularly have fewer colds or flu. This indicates that there may be a direct relationship between getting regular adjustments and the immune system.

Chiropractic patients also tend to sleep better than patients who don't get regular adjustments.

How can chiropractic care promote health in an aging person?

Chiropractic care is great for the aging patient because chiropractic care helps to maintain optimal functioning of the spine and other joints.

The goal of chiropractic care is to improve the function of the spine and other joints and to pump out the inflammation by creating motion in the joints and closing down the pain gates. You want your patients to have optimal function. Much of chiropractic care is about controlling pain and achieving optimum functioning. Pain can lead to other problems, and people with chronic pain are prone to depression.

Once the joints are functioning properly, balance is restored in the body and you function better. For the aging population, when you're able to function and do things on your own, you can take care of yourself and stay in your own home. When you function well, you can be more productive. This is how we can help people with longevity.

Chiropractic care and spinal adjustment can also help with balance issues, which can be a problem as we age as this can lead to falls. A chiropractor can show patients techniques to help with balance, and they can address other areas affecting balance such as ankle function.

Some ways to deal with setbacks?

If an issue or trauma arises you need to start intervention right away. You need to address the injury or condition as soon as it starts. In the event of a trauma, you may want to choose chiropractic or physical therapy.

Degenerating starts after the age of 20 and we all degenerate at different speeds.

How can chiropractic care complement your fitness program?

Chiropractic care and working out are a good combination because it helps you to get more out of your workouts. Professional athletes all use chiropractic care as part of their regular fitness routines.

When you first visit a chiropractor, you should address any existing problems you may have. A chiropractor should do an exam to check range of motion and muscle balance along with alignment. Their goal is to get you functioning better, or so that your joints, nerves and muscles are working optimally.

You have to do things for yourself to keep yourself functioning properly. Exercise is crucial even for people who already have issues, including arthritis, bone loss and other conditions. Regular exercise will help you feel better for longer periods of time.

What kind of exercise is most beneficial if you have bone loss, osteopenia or osteoporosis?

If you have bone loss, or osteoporosis or osteopenia, you don't want to do high intensity activity but do you want to have some weight-bearing exercise because this will help to slow down the bone loss.

Working out in the pool is very beneficial for people with bone loss issues or joint pain and swimming is great for the neuromusculoskeletal system. In the water, you're buoyant, there's resistance, and it works a lot of muscle groups.

Walking is a very underrated activity that almost anyone can do. Generally you don't hurt yourself while walking and you can get a lot of benefits from a fast walk.

You want to make sure you do weight-bearing exercises for that will strengthen all the muscle groups. There's also something to be said about starting out small and doing a little bit at first and then progressing.

It's a good idea to partner with someone. Starting out with a trainer who will teach you how to develop a plan of action is a good first step. Working out with a personal trainer will help you get more from your workouts when you first start because you'll have guidance and you'll be less likely to sustain an injury because you'll be learning the proper technique.

CHAPTER 12

Happily Ever After

At last, you are ready to get started working towards productive longevity, ready to start making your body stronger, more flexible and more fit. You've laced up your sneakers and are all set to break a sweat and be done with it. Stop right there! I'm sure that's probably how you've gone about starting a new exercise program in the past—and because you are a very determined person, it's probably worked okay for a week or two.

There are a couple of typical scenarios. Some people join a gym and immediately begin a program that is too intense, and wind up getting injured. At that point, they're not likely to go back to the gym. Another scenario is the person who starts off exercising every day for a week or two, but hasn't really fully embraced it. You start off walking every single day. But then it rains for three days in a row, so you can't get out and walk. Or you have guests visiting from out of town and so now you have no privacy to do your workout. Or it's Sue's birthday and everyone is taking her out for lunch and you can't resist the fettuccini Alfredo and of course there's the cake once you're back at your desk. Regardless of the reason, you stop working out. You stop being active and watching what you eat, and before you know it, you feel unhealthy, and find yourself discouraged and disappointed.

The best way to avoid this vicious cycle is with knowledge and preparation. Realize that you are not starting another diet to drop a quick 10 pounds. You are making a commitment to yourself to get healthier so that you can stay active and independent for as long as possible. This is a lifestyle makeover, not a month-long routine to get ready for summer.

That's actually good news. What it means is that you can avoid the all-

or-nothing mentality that you may have had with your previous attempts to get fit. This time, you are going to plan the steps you will take and how you will implement them so that you do not get overwhelmed. Doing too much too fast is a sure-fire way to sabotage your chances for success.

If you are a person who is easily overwhelmed, I want you to make one positive change at a time. Start with the exercise routine in Chapter 9. Decide how many days a week you will work out—ideally, I would recommend that you exercise five days a week. This will allow you to break the exercises into groups so that you end up working each muscle group twice each week. Do this for 30 days. That's about half the time researchers have shown that it takes for something to become a habit, but it will give you plenty of time to get comfortable with the idea of working out daily. Then make another positive change, I suggest you revamp your diet after reading Dr. Magoulas' section on Nutrition. Daily exercise and a healthy diet will result in a healthier, fitter body.

Next, consider scheduling an appointment with a chiropractor. The chiropractor will examine you and may make some adjustments to your alignment. You may need several visits to "straighten things out," but having your body properly aligned can make a huge difference in your workout. This will enable you to achieve optimum function, and can make it much easier to maintain proper form throughout the movements.

Find ways to incorporate fitness into your life. Learn a new sport or pick up one you used to play. Schedule a bowling night with your friends. Go for a walk in the park with your spouse or your child. Challenge your grandkids to a Wii tournament. Not only will you be adding social events that are healthy and active, you will be building memories with your friends and family.

Last, but certainly not least, add a spiritual aspect to your life. Regardless of your religion, you can cultivate a connection to the world around you and the force that makes it work. Meditation has been shown to have tremendous capabilities to reduce stress and promote a sense of calm. There are numerous videos and CDs that can lead you through a session.

If meditation seems a bit too much, try simply carving out 10 minutes of solitary, quiet time. Focus on your breathing and the way your body feels as you become healthier and more fit. Practice gratitude and staying in the moment. These things will help slow down your mind and keep you grounded so that you can fully enjoy your life.

Making It Work

If you are the type of person who feels that they have no time to work out, there are several ways you can work in the exercise you need. Some people find they stick to their exercising goals if they schedule their workout times as an appointment. People who are very busy during the day—business owners, busy moms, corporate executives, or even active retirees—find that it helps to fit in a couple of 10 or 20 minute workouts during the day. Especially if you're in front of a computer all day, it's beneficial to get up and move around periodically, so why not fit in a mini workout? There's not one ideal time to exercise, either. If you can only exercise at night after work, then that's when you fit it in. (See my list of Quick Exercises For When You're Strapped For Time in the Appendix.)

Add other changes, perhaps some meditation, schedule some social time with friends, incorporate some physical activity into your weekends—until you have incorporated all the items in your healthy plan and you have designed the life you want.

With a goal of longevity, it is important to realize that you are changing your life. This is not "drop two dress sizes by Memorial Day," and then you can go back to snarfing down junk food in front of the TV. To be active and independent in your 70s, 80s and beyond, you have to start by being active NOW. When you look at the long term goal, three days of rain will not derail your routine—just head back out once the clouds break up. So what if you order the cheesiest, gooiest dinner at Jeffrey's retirement dinner? Resume your sensible food plan the next morning at breakfast.

Moderation is the key to sensible change. Don't start the exercises with weights that are so heavy that you can barely finish the reps. I suggest a weight range for you to begin with, as well as guidelines for determining just how much weight you should begin using for your current ability level. You might have to start out using less weight than I suggest. So what? You need to be comfortable enough to complete the reps using the correct form. Anything more and you run the risk of injury or over-working yourself and burning out. This program is about making steady, consistent and lasting changes in your behavior so that you can see lasting changes in your life.

Celebrate the Changes

Be sure you recognize some of the small changes you will notice along the way. Maybe you'll suddenly realize that you can walk up the stairs without becoming winded, or find that doing bicep curls with eight pound weights are now effortless—be aware of these subtle changes as they are great ways to stay motivated.

Your dietary intake is a key factor, especially if your primary goal is weight loss. You will still see many benefits from incorporating exercise into your life, but if you make dietary changes you will see even more benefits. Eating fresh, high quality food not only gives your body the best possible fuel and top-notch building materials, but it also allows your body to expend more resources on healing itself instead of focusing on digesting highly processed food and neutralizing chemical additives. Making healthy changes to your diet will give you more energy, help you lose more weight and feel better faster.

Don't place all your focus on losing weight. Make sure you incorporate both cardio and strength training into your exercise plan because you need the weight training in order to strengthen your bones. Cardio alone will not be enough. As you build muscle you are stepping up your metabolism. The body reaps an initial caloric burn from the exercising, then more calories are expended as the muscle repairs itself. Finally, there is a higher residual calorie use since muscle tissue requires more energy for basic respiration than fat tissue. This simply means the more fit you become, the easier it is to stay fit–and becoming fit is the goal. "Skinny" or "chubby" are adjectives based on what's fashionable in society. "Fit" on the other hand is a state of being where your body can perform the daily demands placed on it, efficiently and effectively–and that translates into an enhanced quality of life.

Varying your cardio routine will also keep you motivated as it will help to keep your workouts fresh and challenging. Instead of walking or running for every cardio workout, try something new—using the elliptical machine, cycling, rowing, swimming, hiking or dancing are all great cardio exercises. Remember to increase the intensity of your cardio workout over time as you progress so you continue to fully benefit from the exercise.

Finding a sport that you enjoy can make it easier to fit exercise into your life. Even if you've never been a sports-type person, it is never too late to try something new. In fact, learning something new acts as a workout for your brain! Pick a sport that interests you and research it on the internet. Today's technology makes it simple for you to access videos on almost any sport, from archery to Zumba and just about anything in between. Get familiar with the movements, learn the rules—in some cases you will find workout routines so you can prepare for a specific sport by strengthening specific muscles. Take some lessons, if applicable. You can always turn to an expert for advice. Join a club so you meet people who are active in that sport. In my experience, people are usually more than willing to help a novice learn something they enjoy.

In your initial phase of your fitness program, you may need education and some guidance to build your foundation. I am also accessible through my own websites and via e-mail if you ever have any questions or need any clarifications or ideas. If you're in the Central New Jersey area, I can even be available for a consultation.

Congratulations on beginning your journey to productive longevity! I'm certain you will find it a worthwhile and enriching experience.

References

1. http://dictionary.reference.com/browse/personal+trainer?r=66 Last accessed 3/12/2013.
2. http://dictionary.cambridge.org/dictionary/british/personal-trainer Last accessed 3/12/2013.
3. U.S. Department of Health and Human Services. "Healthy People: The Surgeon General's Report on Health Promotion and Disease Prevention." Rockville, MD: U.S. Department of Health and Human Services, Office of the Surgeon General, 1979. Last accessed June 5, 2013. <http://profiles.nlm.nih.gov/NN/B/B/G/K/_/nnbbgk.pdf>.
4. U.S. Department of Health and Human Services. "Bone Health and Osteoporosis: A Report of the Surgeon General." Rockville, MD: U.S. Department of Health and Human Services, Office of the Surgeon General, 2004. <http://www.surgeongeneral.gov/library/reports/bonehealth/full_report.pdf>
5. Centers for Disease Control and Prevention. Injury Prevention & Control: Home & Recreational Safety. "Hip Fractures Among Older Adults." Last accessed June 17, 2013. <http://www.cdc.gov/homeandrecreationalsafety/falls/adulthipfx.html>
6. Centers for Disease Control and Prevention. Injury Prevention & Control: Home & Recreational Safety. "Hip Fractures Among Older Adults." Last accessed June 17, 2013. <http://www.cdc.gov/homeandrecreationalsafety/falls/adulthipfx.html>
7. Centers for Disease Control and Prevention. Diabetes Public Health Resource. "Basics About Diabetes." Last accessed June 17, 2013. <http://www.cdc.gov/diabetes/consumer/learn.htm>
8. Centers for Disease Control and Prevention. Diabetes Public Health Resource. "Prevent Diabetes." Last accessed June 17, 2013. <http://www.cdc.gov/diabetes/consumer/prevent.htm>
9. Centers for Disease Control and Prevention. Diabetes Public Health Resource. "Prevent Diabetes." Last accessed June 17, 2013. <http://www.cdc.gov/diabetes/consumer/prevent.htm>
10. U.S. Department of Health and Human Services. National Institutes of Health, National Institute on Aging. "Healthy Aging: Lessons from the Baltimore Longitudinal Study of Aging." Last accessed June 18, 2013. <http://www.nia.nih.gov/sites/default/files/healthy_aging_lessons_from_the_baltimore_longitudinal_study_of_aging.pdf>
11. U.S. Department of Health and Human Services. National Institutes of Health, National Institute on Aging. "Healthy Aging: Lessons from the Baltimore Longitudinal Study of Aging." Last accessed June 18, 2013. <http://www.nia.nih.gov/sites/default/files/healthy_aging_lessons_from_the_baltimore_longitudinal_study_of_aging.pdf>
12. U.S. Department of Health and Human Services. National Institutes of Health, National Institute on Aging. "Healthy Aging: Lessons from the Baltimore Longitudinal Study of Aging." Last accessed June 18, 2013. <http://www.nia.nih.gov/sites/default/files/healthy_aging_lessons_from_the_baltimore_longitudinal_study_of_aging.pdf>

13. U.S. Dept of Health & Human Services, National Institutes of Health. National Institute on Aging. "Preventing Alzheimer's Disease: What Do We Know?." Last accessed June 20, 2013.
<http://www.nia.nih.gov/sites/default/files/preventing_alzheimers_disease_0.pdf>

14. U.S. Dept of Health & Human Services, National Institutes of Health. National Institute on Aging. "Preventing Alzheimer's Disease: What Do We Know?." Last accessed June 20, 2013.
<http://www.nia.nih.gov/sites/default/files/preventing_alzheimers_disease_0.pdf>

15. U.S. Dept of Health & Human Services, National Institutes of Health. National Institute on Aging. "Preventing Alzheimer's Disease: What Do We Know?." Last accessed June 20, 2013.
<http://www.nia.nih.gov/sites/default/files/preventing_alzheimers_disease_0.pdf>

16. U.S. Dept of Health & Human Services, National Institutes of Health. National Institute on Aging. "Preventing Alzheimer's Disease: What Do We Know?." Last accessed June 20, 2013.
<http://www.nia.nih.gov/sites/default/files/preventing_alzheimers_disease_0.pdf>

17. U.S. Department of Health and Human Services. "Healthy People: The Surgeon General's Report on Health Promotion and Disease Prevention." Rockville, MD: U.S. Department of Health and Human Services, Office of the Surgeon General, 1979. Last accessed June 5, 2013. <http://profiles.nlm.nih.gov/NN/B/B/G/K/_/nnbbgk.pdf>.

18. U.S. Department of Health and Human Services. "Healthy People: The Surgeon General's Report on Health Promotion and Disease Prevention." Rockville, MD: U.S. Department of Health and Human Services, Office of the Surgeon General, 1979. Last accessed June 8, 2013. <http://profiles.nlm.nih.gov/NN/B/B/G/K/_/nnbbgk.pdf>.

19. U.S. Department of Health and Human Services. National Institutes of Health, National Institute on Aging. "Healthy Aging: Lessons from the Baltimore Longitudinal Study of Aging." Last accessed June 18, 2013.
<http://www.nia.nih.gov/sites/default/files/healthy_aging_lessons_from_the_baltimore_longitudinal_study_of_aging.pdf>

20. U.S. Department of Health and Human Services. National Institutes of Health, National Institute on Aging. "Healthy Aging: Lessons from the Baltimore Longitudinal Study of Aging." Last accessed June 18, 2013.
<http://www.nia.nih.gov/sites/default/files/healthy_aging_lessons_from_the_baltimore_longitudinal_study_of_aging.pdf>

21. U.S. Department of Health and Human Services. National Institutes of Health, National Institute on Aging. "Healthy Aging: Lessons from the Baltimore Longitudinal Study of Aging." Last accessed June 18, 2013.
<http://www.nia.nih.gov/sites/default/files/healthy_aging_lessons_from_the_baltimore_longitudinal_study_of_aging.pdf>

APPENDIX:

CHECKLISTS & QUICKSTARTS

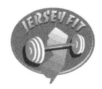

Self-Assessment of Fitness Level

Weight: _____   Height: _____

Measurements: Chest: _____ Waist: _____ Hips: _____

                Upper Arm: _____ Thigh: _____ Calf: _____

Clothing Size: _____

Blood Pressure: _____

Resting Pulse Rate: _____

Number of sit-ups possible: _____

Number of push-ups possible: _____

How many flights of stairs can you climb before getting winded? _____

How long can you maintain the Plank pose? _____

Ten Questions to Help Determine Your Fitness Goals

1) Do I want to improve my overall appearance or just focus on certain parts of my body?

2) Do I have any physical skills I want to improve or enhance?

3) Is my goal to build endurance, flexibility or strength or all three?

4) Is my goal strictly to lose weight?

5) Are my expectations realistic?

6) Do I want to make a lifestyle change?

7) Do I have a specific deadline for this goal?

8) Should I seek the services of a professional?

9) When was the last time I had a physical and is it time to go in for another one?

10) Am I mentally ready to make a change?

Eraldo's 8 Quick Changes To Improve Your Diet and Health

1. Eliminate all deep fried foods from your diet. Try foods that are steamed or broiled instead.

2. Do an inventory of your refrigerator and pantry to see what kind of healthy foods you usually have on hand. Try some new healthy foods.

3. Instead of eliminating foods, try cutting calories through portion control. This is something you can do even when you're eating at home by eating on a smaller plate.

4. Increase your intake of fruits and vegetables. Aim for five servings a day.

5. Get rid of sugary drinks – there is no room for these in a healthy diet. Even fruit juices are very high in sugar. Drinking water or unsweetened tea are better choices. You should also limit diet sodas as well.

6. Limit your intake of white sugar and processed sugar.

7. Stop smoking immediately.

8. Moderate your consumption of alcohol.

Quick Exercises When You're Strapped for Time

Strengthen your muscles when you're on the go with these quick exercises. Complete a few sets before you head out the door, when you get home from work or even at the office.

1. Dips: Put two sturdy chairs together a little more than shoulder width apart. Place yourself in an upright position with your hands on the chairs without letting your feet touch the floor. Bend your elbows to a 90 degree angle. Push yourself back to the upright position.

2. Pull-ups: Invest in a workout bar to do pull-ups. Workout bars are portable and easy to use—just find a door frame to place it on and you're ready to go.

3. Sit-ups and crunches: You can do sit-ups and crunches right on the floor or use a stability ball. While you're not using the stability ball for core exercises, you can use it as a chair at your desk. It's great for keeping good posture.

4. Hip extensions: Strengthen the hamstring and gluteus muscles by doing hip extensions with a resistance band. Tie one end of the band around something sturdy at ankle height and tie the other end around your ankle. Shift all your weight to the leg without the band. Keep your body stable and straighten the leg with the band behind you. Return to the starting position.

5. Jump rope: You can burn over 100 calories in 10 minutes by jumping rope. Find an area with space, grab your jump rope and start jumping!

It's never too late to start integrating fitness into your life. There's always time to get in a workout or even just a few exercises. You really don't need more than 30-40 minutes a day to achieve your fitness goals. Make the most of your training time by focusing on your objectives. Your health is just as important as your career or any other aspect in your life, so try to make it a priority.

Cardio on the Run

Throughout this book I have given you lots of examples of sports and activities that will provide you with a cardio workout. There are numerous things you can do which will increase your heart rate enough to be in the training zone to qualify as "cardio." But perhaps you are travelling and don't have access to your tennis partner or your aerobics class. What then?

For those of you who don't really care about a specific sport, or need something easy and portable that will still deliver results, I recommend running. You simply can't get more basic than running—unless it's walking, but it's tricky to keep the heart rate high enough for a long enough time to burn a significant amount of calories when walking. So, running it is. Here's a few tips to get started.

Educate. Go to the library or online and read about running. There are plenty of sources to teach you the basic stride, and everything from how your foot should hit the ground to how to train for a marathon. Determine the terrain you will be running on most often—pavement, cinder, dirt, grass?

Equipment. Go to a running store or other athletic store and buy a good pair of shoes. Since shoes are the primary equipment for this activity, it is essential that they fit properly and enhance your performance. Tell the store staff what surface you will mostly be running on and give them an estimate of how many miles per week. Will you be jogging or sprinting? They should analyze your gait and pick the shoe that works best for you.

I suggest you also invest in a heart rate monitor watch. Some devices today not only monitor your heart rate but serve as a stopwatch and a pedometer as well. Take advantage of this technology! There is a smartphone app that will track your route and share it on the internet. If it helps to motivate you, do it!

Environment. Decide where you will run. Inside on the treadmill? Outdoors in the park or just around the neighborhood? Again, plan your route so that you are motivated to get out there every day. But be sensible. Don't run alone in an isolated area. Try not to run at night or in an unfamiliar neighborhood. Safety is more important than maintaining your routine!

Enjoyment. Many people find that having a running buddy helps by keeping you accountable and for bringing a bit of a social aspect to your routine. Start slow—if you have been essentially sedentary then you might want to begin by alternating jogging and walking. Progress by increasing the jogging intervals and decreasing the walking portions. As you get proficient, find a path with more hills or if indoors, increase the intensity on the treadmill. Set a goal, whether it is to run a 5K race or just to jog all the way around the block without stopping. Having something to strive for lends a challenge to your workout and can be a motivating factor. Celebrate when you reach your goal, and be sure to track your progress.

Although certain health concerns will need close monitoring, such as knee issues, running is one sport that is basically accessible to everyone. It is easy, cheap and convenient—and therefore an excellent cardio workout for a beginner.

ACKNOWLEDGMENTS

They say that behind every successful man there is a more successful woman, and then more.

I would like to acknowledge my family first of all—my wife Lina, daughter Francesca and son Robert. They are my life and without them I wouldn't have a reason to move forward. My dad, Eraldo Maglara Sr., and my mom, Emma Maglara. Their love and support have made me the man I am today.

To my sister, Captain Patrizia Maglara, USA, retired, you are my hero. I am so proud of you for dedicating your life to protect this wonderful country we live in. I will always have a special place in my heart for you.

To my sister Ellen and my brother Alex: I always felt like a "second" father figure to both of you. I am thankful for all of the wonderful memories we have shared and for the new ones still to be had. I am blessed to have you both in my life.

A special thanks to many others who have been a major influence: Jerry and Laura Bove, Luigi and Cindy Bove, Robert and Mellisa Bove and Giuseppe and Sonia Bove.

To my mother-in-law Clara Bove. Your love, caring and tenacity have always inspired me to be the best that I can be—I've learned so much from you.

And finally to my best friend Marco Tedeschi for always being there for me.

I would also like to acknowledge all the professionals who were instrumental in creating this book. Special thanks to Mary Ellen and Stacy from The Write Room, LLC, my terrific writing and editing team. Alan Leckner of Leckner Design Associates, for his artistic contributions and for helping me bring these exercises to life. Photographer Alyse Liebowitz of 3 Chicks That Click Photography for her vision and the wonderful images that came from it.

I want to thank Dr. Larry Arbeitman, DC and Dr. Sharon Barnum, DC for their time and expertise, and to Dr. Steven Lisser, MD for his excellent introduction. A special thanks to Dr. Lori Magoulas, PhD, for sharing her comprehensive knowledge of nutrition and her insights.

And my gratitude for the tireless efforts of Jen and Danielle of InBloom Communications for publicizing my endeavors.

I'd like to thank all my clients whose hard work is an inspiration to me every day. I look forward to sharing in your continued success.

ABOUT THE AUTHOR

Eraldo Maglara is a graduate of the National Personal Training Institute and is a certified personal trainer with the National Strength and Conditioning Association. He is the owner and operator of Fitness Training by Eraldo, Inc., in Marlboro, New Jersey. His personal training clients include men and women, ranging from busy moms and corporate executives to retirees.

Maglara's personal training practice has been featured in a number of regional publications and news outlets, including In Jersey Magazine and the Asbury Park Press. He blogs about health and fitness on his websites, JerseyFitTv.com, EraldoFitness.com, and TheRealFountainOfYouthBook.com and has been a contributing author for a number of publications.

Maglara is an active member of a number of Central New Jersey business and professional associations. For several years, he has served as a board member of the Matawan-Aberdeen Chamber of Commerce. He is a graduate of Richard Stockton University, and holds a Bachelor's Degree in Business.

He lives in Marlboro, New Jersey with his wife and two children.

About Stacy Reagan and Mary Ellen Landolfi

Stacy Reagan and Mary Ellen Landolfi have been collaborating on writing projects since they were undergraduate students at Drew University in Madison, New Jersey. They are the founders and co-owners of The Write Room, LLC., a New Jersey writing and editorial services company. Collectively, they are involved in a number of business and professional organizations including the American Medical Writers Association, Liberty States Fiction Writers, Navesink Business Group, New Jersey Association of Women Business Owners and the Northern Monmouth Chamber of Commerce.

They would like to thank Eraldo Maglara for this incredible opportunity and their families for their support as they continue their writing and entrepreneurial adventures.

IF you enjoyed this book,
please consider posting a review at Amazon.
It would be greatly appreciated.

Fitness Training by Eraldo

www.EraldoFitness.com

We specialize in "in-home" personal training. We get results, period... and this is how we do it:

1. We design a program that's tailored just for you... not the general public!

2. We will educate and guide you on the right path to dieting and nutrition.

3. Our fitness software will record and track your progress every week – so you can see the results!

4. No equipment – no problem! We bring everything to you, saving you money on bulky and expensive equipment.

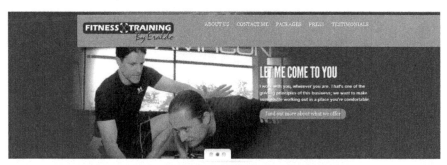

What's your biggest fitness problem? Let Eraldo help you achieve your goals

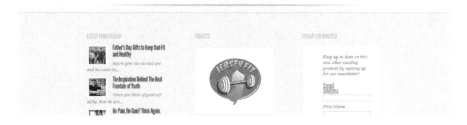

Here's what Eraldo's clients are saying:

"I put off getting in shape for so long because I was nervous about going into a gym. When I found Eraldo, I knew that he was exactly what I needed. He got me into the best shape of my life!" Joan A.

"I don't run. But I'm taking a police test that requires running. I called Eraldo and within 3 weeks, I was able run 30-minutes non-stop. Call Eraldo. His methods work." Dan S.

Visit www.EraldoFitness.com regularly to catch up on his newest blog posts and other updates.

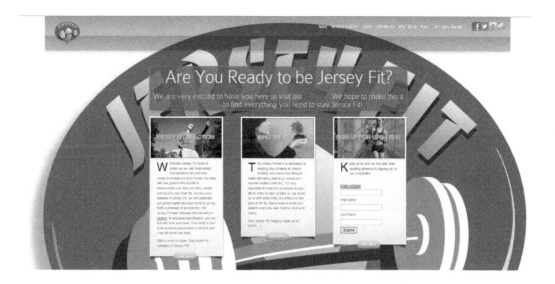

Are you ready to be Jersey Fit?

The Jersey Fit team is dedicated to helping you achieve an overall healthy and stress-free lifestyle, while still being able to go about your normal routine each day. It's very important to maintain a balance in your life in order to stay healthy but for some of us with busy lives, it's difficult to find time to do so. We're here to show you simple ways you can improve your well-being.

Jersey Fit, Inc. founder and Certified Personal Trainer Eraldo Maglara provides fitness expertise and practical tips and ideas through his website, blog and in his fitness and exercise videos.

For the latest updates, visit www.JerseyFitTV.com

CPSIA information can be obtained at www.ICGtesting.com
Printed in the USA
BVOW10s1851290615

406688BV00008B/70/P